Clean Slate

C L E A N S E

WORKBOOK

LINDSEY ELMORE, Pharm D, BCPS

CLEAN SLATE CLEANSE: Workbook

© 2019 by Lindsey Elmore

All Rights Reserved

ISBN 978-1-7336028-0-8

ISBN (eBook) 978-1-7336028-1-5

Design and Layout: Shelbi Kribell

Photography: Justin Anderson and Shelbi Kribell

Recipe Testing and Editing: Samantha McKenzie

Editor: Jen McCraw

Published in the United States.

A LINDSEY KAY ELMORE BOOK

PRAISE FOR THE CLEANSE FROM PREVIOUS CLEANSERS

The Cleanse taught me that I'm strong enough. That I have the willpower to accomplish everything I want, I just need to forget about fear.

DANIELA H

The Cleanse helped reset my relationship with food, and I more clearly see food as nutrition for my body and not just for the taste buds.

TAMMY G

I joined to see what the plan would be and found this cleanse is built for success. Everything is mapped out right down to the grocery list.

GAIL P

I lost a total of 13 lbs....I didn't do this cleanse for weight loss but it's only a plus! I feel so much better as far as energy levels go and just in general. I've been on medication for chronic headaches and migraines for quite some time. I think gluten was the culprit! I am actually going to continue eating this way except I will be enjoying my 1 cup of coffee in the morning.

DENISE K

Lost weight in areas I always struggle losing weight. My sleep has never been this amazing! I plan to add in some things back to my diet, but I'm feeling and looking great and I intend to keep it that way. Lifestyle change.

SHELBI K

Eating mindfully revealed that I often eat more than I need to and too fast. As I became more conscious of the feeling of having enough, I was able to be fully satisfied with less and not feeling "stuffed". I also am enjoying my food more, not just trying to get it over with. The cleanse taught me to be more aware of my body signals, eating only when I am hungry, eating slowly so the body has time to process and signal when full.

MARIA T

I am SUPER STOKED with my results and LOVED every bit of this Cleanse!!!

SHAWNA A

TABLE OF CONTENTS

To mom, for feeding me even when I didn't want to eat.

FOREWORD

When I first began my health and wellness journey, I was plagued by eczema that I was convinced would never heal. Through my autoimmune disorders, I set myself up on a path where I began to travel the world in search of naturally healing foods, ingredients, cultural wellness traditions, and science. I discovered the key to wellness came from within, and is impacted by how and what we eat, how we move and even how we practice self-care.

After being introduced to Lindsey, I became so inspired by her wellness journey. She started her dive into wellness due to a toxic relationship with food and decided to craft her own approach to recovery. As a young woman with bulimia, Lindsey had beaten herself up with food day after day. Subsiding on sugar and caffeine, ended up leading her to depression, self-doubt, and a deep-seeded anger. She became a vegetarian, not to sustain a healthy lifestyle, but to further restrict what she would allow herself to eat.

Much like me, her journey shifted when she first encountered an acupuncturist during her time in pharmacy school. As my own journey of discovery lead me to become immersed in the science and impact of autophagy (our body's own cellular detox process) on our health, Lindsey became immersed in Chinese medicine's interpretation of health. Lindsey was raised in a very Western medicine environment. The daughter of a nurse, she thought health was simply a lack of disease, and that when disease existed, it was simply a matter of finding the right drug to fix the problem. Due to Lindsey's exposure to Chinese medicine - herbs, tinctures, and food became her primary source of health.

Lindsey had always loved to cook, but living in San Francisco broadened her horizons, and introduced her to new ethnic cuisines. Instead of the dairy-rich casseroles, meat-focused plates, and sugar-laden desserts of her childhood, Lindsey turned to spices, organic and locally sourced foods, and taught herself to love vegetables that she swore she would never eat.

Because of her new-found passion, Lindsey developed a two-part cleanse cookbook/workbook to introduce readers to a refreshing yet simple plan to begin a healthy lifestyle. Lindsey's The Clean Slate Cleanse Cookbook is packed with flavorful recipes that reflect Lindsey's life, from vegan makeovers of traditional soul foods like the Black-Eyed Peas and Collard Greens she ate as a child on New Year's Day, to dishes like Thai Green Curry and Tofu Makhani, that reflect her extensive travel and ever-expanding palate. The Clean Slate Cleanse has a recipe for everyone!

Whereas, Lindsey's cookbook focuses on the recipes, The Clean Slate Cleanse Workbook offers transforming daily routines, and intentionally seeks to support individuals in becoming more mindful of what they eat. The difference from this cleanse is that there is so much more than just science: there is yoga, journaling, mindful eating exercises, and daily trackers that can assess individual progress. The Workbook takes what could be a difficult dietary transition and transforms it into a daily discipline that can be accomplished with ease.

Lindsey hosted her first vegan cleanse back in 2009 for a small group of friends. In the past two years, she has lead hundreds of people through what is now the Clean Slate Cleanse. I am proud of Lindsey for positioning herself as a flexitarian. She doesn't claim to be vegan all the time, and in fact freely admits that her initial go at vegetarianism was anything but the pursuit of health. She loves a good glass of wine occasionally, but during the cleanse, Lindsey leads a team with discipline, love, and determination.

Dr. Lindsey Elmore is nothing short of brilliant and The Clean Slate Cleanse is nothing short of life changing! Lindsey makes science simple, understandable and inspires individuals to care for themselves by instilling confidence in them.

- Naomi Whittel, Author of Glow15

INTRODUCTION

Let me start by saying this: I am not vegan all the time. I drink alcohol and caffeine, eat gluten and sugar occasionally as well. Before you throw this book to the side, understand that even though I do eat in ways that are different than this cleanse, I do it mindfully. I take inventory of what I am eating. What is in it? Where did it come from? How does my mind feel about it? How does my body feel? Do my mind and body feel the same? I also take at least two times per year to cleanse. I find that it changes my palate, boosts my metabolism, and helps me to maintain body weight. It also helps reinforce better eating decisions on a regular basis.

Some may say that it is inauthentic for me to write this book without being 100% committed to all the suggestions that are in here, but I disagree. I have been completing dietary cleanses since 2009, and since then I've read more about the mind-food connection, worked with healers who help you to stay present in the body from day to day, and trained extensively in essential oils as a tool to release clogged up emotions. From all of these learnings, I created the Clean Slate Cleanse.

I recommend cleansing for a few reasons:

1. We live in a world where time and space seem to swirl around us. We grab a quick sandwich, a cheeky glass of wine, or a dessert without quite thinking about it. We sit and eat an entire plate of food without enjoying it, or struggle to choke our food down over an angry conversation with a loved one. Cleansing creates a necessary purposefulness with food and resets us back to baseline.
2. We fall into traps with food. We can lose our sense of adventure in favor of the same old dishes that we always eat. Cleansing offers an opportunity to explore new items on the menu and invite new vibrancy and health to us.
3. We lean too heavily on supplements and medicines. Seriously, eating a terrible diet will trump any supplement or medicine every single time.
4. There is very strong, albeit debatable and contested, evidence that plant-based diets are the healthiest way to eat both for our bodies and our planet. I will review this topic throughout the book, and you can decide for yourself. I have confidence that consumption of meat and animal products is (at least) unnecessary for humans and (at worst) harmful to humans.
5. As a woman who recovered from bulimia, I find that cleansing reminds me to use food to nourish and empower my body, instead of using food to abuse my body.
6. Just because, darn it, you feel better, your skin is clearer, and your belly is flatter.

Whether this way of eating becomes a lifestyle choice or a temporary break, it is nice to know that we have options to reclaim our relationship with food. This cleanse eliminates meat and animal products, gluten, most sugars, caffeine, and alcohol for 21 days. Thankfully there are hundreds of delicious plants to eat on the cleanse, and the list of plant-based and gluten-free prepared foods has expanded extensively over the past few years. I understand that this style of eating can cost more up front, especially if it is a dramatic overhaul. However, once you get going, the ingredients in your made-over pantry will be used over and over again.

I hate the word *diet*. This cleanse is not intended to be a set of restrictions that prevent you from experiencing pleasure from food, nor is it intended to be a "Phew, thank God that horrid diet is over, so I can go back to cakes and coffee after my steak". This book is intended to reset your brain to the original definition of the word diet: from the 13th century, a noun meaning "regular food, the kind of food that a person, animal or community normally eats". Never in this book do I use the word diet as a verb meaning "to restrict oneself to small amounts or special kinds of food to lose weight". The purpose of this cleanse is not to lose weight, but to examine and explore our relationship with food. To look at the regular food we eat and determine if it is serving our body to live at its maximum potential.

There are two books in this series: The *Clean Slate Cleanse Cookbook* and the *Clean Slate Cleanse Workbook.* The cookbook is exactly that: more than 100 plant-based recipes for breakfast, lunch, dinner, snack, juices, and pantry staples. This workbook is a day to day guide for the Clean Slate Cleanse. You can track your progress, get inspiration, complete a daily exercise, and reflect on your journey. There is also a sample meal plan in the workbook. If you choose to follow the meal plan, then pay special attention to the weekly and daily food prep advice to save time in the kitchen.

If you're doing this cleanse alone, it can be tough. Join one of our live cleanses and get the support of a community of #cleanslaters, access to a private Facebook education group and inspirational Marco Polo group, and complete the cleanse live with me! I'd love to see you there! Head to www.lindseyelmore.com/cleanse to get started!

Sending you so much love! Blessings on your Clean Slate Cleanse journey!

Lindsey Elmore

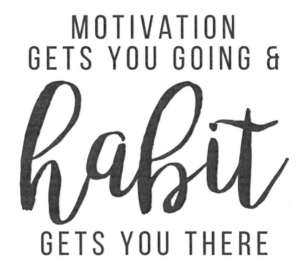

MOTIVATION
GETS YOU GOING &
habit
GETS YOU THERE

- ZIG ZIGLAR -

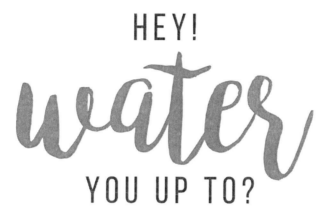

HEY! water YOU UP TO?

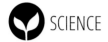 # SCIENCE

Let's start out by talking about how to make life easier on a cleanse. People often give up on a cleanse like this one because it can seem challenging to do this day after day. It takes resolve to choose the salad with oil and vinegar when everyone else is eating a hamburger at a restaurant.

Preparation is one of your best weapons in the armament of defense against failure. Our entire life is simply a compilation of our habits, and in order to change our lives, we must change our habits.[1] Let's talk through a few top tips to make this easier on you.

BRING YOUR FRIENDS AND FAMILY

Life is more fun with friends! While you must find your own dedication, sharing this journey with your friends and family can make it a much more enjoyable experience. With a friend, you can share your victories and failures, as well as new recipes and experiences. If you are about to start the cleanse on your own, think of 10 friends who might be open to joining along with you and call each of them. Also, be clear to people in your household that you will complete the cleanse and invite them to join with you. The Clean Slate Cleanse is much easier when everyone in your house is on board for at least the meals you share together.

CHOOSE NEW CONVENIENT FOODS

Instead of chips, candies or cheese, slice and dice vegetables such as cucumber, carrot, celery, and zucchini and have dipping sauces such as hummus, vegan salad dressing, and guacamole on hand. Keep convenient snacks available to make it easier to make simple, positive decisions between meals.

CLEAN OUT THE PANTRY

The easiest and simplest way to avoid unhealthy eating is to avoid bringing unhealthy food into your home. Clean out as many of the non cleanse-approved foods as possible so you don't grab for them in a moment of hunger.

CREATE A BANK OF STAPLE INGREDIENTS

Go ahead and cook rice, quinoa, and beans for quick incorporation into recipes. If you are following the suggested meal plan, you will find that some days are prep days for the week to come. For example, days 0, 7, and 14 require a lot of cooking, but it will make life so much easier for you the rest of the week. In the recipe section, I have included a selection of my favorite pantry staple recipes. Simply having these in your refrigerator will help you cook meals quickly throughout the cleanse.

LEARN YOUR LEFTOVERS

In my house, almost every dish I cook becomes a leftover meal. In fact, I like to think of these as *next*overs. Vegan food makes the easiest toppings for salad the next day for lunch. Keep vegetable stock on hand, and you can easily turn rice dishes into soup the next day. Breakfast tofu scramble can easily be made into a wrap for a delicious lunch. Finding new ways to use leftovers prevents food waste and saves your precious energy in the kitchen.

SHOP WITH EASE

The number of vegan, gluten-free, and sugar-free options at the grocery store has extensively expanded in the past few years. Ingredients that used to be obscure and difficult to source can be found at corner stores. You can find sections dedicated to specialty diets even at regular conventional grocery stores. Specialty grocers are in a ton of different locations these days, and this can also make finding ingredients easier. Maybe take a trip to the store just to explore and take inventory of what is there before starting on the cleanse.

The availability of food ingredients found for little to no shipping at online retailers has exploded over the past few years. From Amazon Fresh to meal box delivery services like Purple Carrot, it is now easier than ever to find ways to eat according to the cleanse. If you can't find an ingredient in a store, be sure to check online. Spend some time getting to know your local resources, as well as online, to find quick and easy sources for food.

DINING OUT ON THE CLEANSE

If you have access to great vegan cuisine in your town, then you are in luck! If not, it is very likely that you will go out to eat with people who eat meat, dairy, sugar, gluten, and drink alcohol during your cleanse. You must be ready to see what is on the menu and order wisely with pride. There are many people who will actively oppose this style of eating, and that is okay. You are strong, happy, and healthy, and fully empowered to complete this cleanse. When reviewing a standard menu, here are a few options and adaptations:

1. Salads without cheese or meat. Choose dressing that is oil-based; oil and vinegar is the safest choice, as many bottled vinaigrettes contain sugar.
2. Soups. Many menus will denote if a soup is vegetarian, but you may still have to ask about cream or butter. Tomato-based broth soups without meat or pasta seem to be some of the safest choices.
3. Sides. Check for options like steamed broccoli, asparagus, green beans, or carrots. Roasted sweet potatoes, Brussels sprouts, or mushrooms may also be an option, as long as there is no butter added. There may be undisclosed meat in the sides, and you may choose to ask your server for advice.
4. If you are at a nicer restaurant, you may be able to ask the chef to make a vegan plate.

CHILL OUT WITH THE FIRST GROCERY SHOP

I am not going to lie, the first trip to the grocery store after making a dietary change like this one can be expensive and time consuming. But I promise you the ingredients will repeat time and time again throughout the cleanse.

BE SURE TO READ THE RECIPE IN ADVANCE

Some of the recipes in this book take preparation, even overnight preparation. Therefore, it is very important to read the entire recipe before starting to cook. I also highly recommend completing all slicing, dicing, and portioning before beginning to cook.

EMBRACE THE SUCCESS AND STRUGGLE

Let's just go ahead and accept that every single day on this cleanse is not going to be easy. Struggling through a day is okay; we all go through struggles. Keep your chin up. Remember your daily mantras, and just go one bite of food at a time.

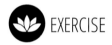 EXERCISE

To make the transition into the cleanse easy, let's start with water. Water can really help you to adjust for the potential sugar and caffeine crash that may be ahead. Every day on the cleanse, you will have the opportunity to track your water intake. I very strongly encourage you to crush at least eight 8 oz. glasses of water per day and even more if you are exercising, breastfeeding, or in a hot environment where you are sweating. This can help you avoid headaches, flush toxins, and keep your head clear as you go through the cleanse.

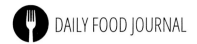 DAILY FOOD JOURNAL

Before we begin, let's talk about what foods we do and don't eat on the cleanse. With the Clean Slate Cleanse, we are eliminating most sugar, all alcohol, animal products, gluten, and caffeine. You may be wondering what exactly you will be eating, and there are so many options. Recently there has been an explosion in the number of vegan and gluten-free prepared foods. But buyer beware! Read the labels closely to avoid sugars.

Below is a list of foods that you can eat at any point during the cleanse, and some foods that are better left at the store. Be creative! Try new foods, and have fun doing it. Remember: don't dial in on the cleanse and just eat tortillas packed with vegan cheese every day. Focus on vegetables, beans, legumes, and whole foods. For some of my favorite brands of foods, check out Appendix 4.

FOODS TO BRING INTO THE CLEANSE

- Aquafaba: the juice from chickpeas that can be used to bind and cream ingredients. Save your juice from chickpea recipes as it can be used as an egg substitute.
- Beans and legumes: adzuki beans, black beans, black-eyed peas, chickpeas, edamame, fava beans, lentils, lima beans, peanuts, and soy beans. Dried beans are best because the end-product is tastier when cooked correctly, but they must be soaked in advance and do take a while to cook. Canned beans and legumes are also fine and offer a quick and convenient option.
- Bread: gluten-free bread, buns, and tortillas (ensure that they are egg-free and non-GMO).
- Butter (vegan): Use caution as many vegan butters are full of additives and GMO ingredients. Earth Balance is a brand easily found. A lot of people choose to avoid vegan butter as it is a type of margarine, albeit cleaner than the hydrogenated stuff. You can always use oil instead.
- Cheeses, vegan varieties: almond, aquafaba, cashew, soy, tofu, or vegetable (preferably rennet- and casein-free).
- Corn chips: non-GMO. (Be careful here; you can eat a lot of corn chips on this type of eating plan.)
- Corn grits and polenta: non-GMO.
- Crackers and cakes: almond, flax, nut, rice, and seed crackers and cakes.
- Faux meats: burgers, sausage patties, "meat crumbles," "chicken" patties. Make sure all are gluten-free. (Use caution here. Some of these faux meats can be very unhealthy. Ensure that they are non-GMO and do not contain added sugars. It is better to focus on getting vegetables versus training yourself that meat or a meat substitute is necessary at each meal).
- Flours: gluten-free, such as arrowroot, bean, buckwheat, chickpea, nut, pea, potato, rice, seed, soy, and tapioca.

- Fruits: apples, avocados, bananas, blueberries, cherries, goji berries, figs, grapefruit, lemons, limes, oranges, peaches, pears, and frozen fruits for smoothies. Most fruits are acceptable; avoid high glycemic index fruits (see below).
- Grains: amaranth, Arborio rice, basmati rice, black rice, brown rice, buckwheat, corn (non-GMO), jasmine rice, millet, quinoa, teff, white rice, and wild rice.
- Guacamole: make your own or buy from store.
- Herbal teas: chamomile, peppermint, rooibos, vanilla spice, or any other naturally decaffeinated herbal tea.
- Hummus: make your own (see recipes in the *CSC Cookbook* on pp. 98 – 101) or buy from store.
- Juices: pomegranate, cranberry juice for sparkling-water cocktails, vegetable juices (unsweetened).
- Mayonnaise (vegan): make your own, see recipes in the *CSC Cookbook* pp. 38 – 40, or find store brands.
- Milk: non-dairy almond, cashew, coconut, hemp, rice, or soy milk (unsweetened).
- Mixed-grain hot cereals: be sure they're gluten- and sugar-free.
- Mushrooms: button, cremini, hen of the woods, miatake, portobello, shiitake, etc.
- Nut or seed butters: almond butter, cashew butter, peanut butter, tahini, (all sugar-free).
- Nuts: almonds, brazil nuts, cashews, filberts, macadamia nuts, pecans, pistachios, walnuts, etc.
- Oats: Irish steel-cut and old-fashioned gluten-free oats.
- Oils (plant-based): avocado, canola (non-GMO), coconut, flaxseed, olive (extra-virgin), sesame, sunflower and safflower (high-oleic versions), walnut, etc. Use caution not to overuse as oils can dramatically increase fat and saturated fat content. These can be added to vegetable juices and smoothies to diversify the nutrient content and prevent blood sugar spikes.
- Pasta: amaranth, artichoke, buckwheat, chickpea, corn (non-GMO), lentil, potato, or quinoa, rice, or tofu.
- Pasta: gluten-free amaranth, buckwheat, chickpea, rice, etc.
- Popcorn: non-GMO.
- Protein powder: non-dairy hemp, pea, rice, or soy based.
- Rice wrappers: Asian style.
- Salsas: tomato, mango, pineapple, or other fruit salsas.
- Seasonings: garlic, ginger, Himalayan pink or Celtic sea salt, liquid aminos, Maldon salt, pepper, tamari, all herbs, both fresh and dried.
- Seeds: chia, flax, hemp, pumpkin, sesame, sunflower, etc.
- Stock: vegetarian soup base, or vegetable bullion.
- Sweeteners: agave nectar, brazzein, coconut sugar, curculin, guo, inulin, luo han miraculin, monellin, monkfruit sugar, pentadin, stevia, yacon syrup, and other natural sugars with a glycemic index less than 35. Avoid as often as possible.
- Tempeh: (non-GMO).

- Tofu: (non-GMO).
- Tortillas: unsweetened, non-GMO buckwheat, corn or rice.
- Vegetables: artichokes, arugula, asparagus, broccoli, Brussels sprouts, carrots, cauliflower, collard greens, cucumbers, eggplant, endive, escarole, garlic, green beans, kale, mixed greens, mustard greens, peas, radicchio, radishes, romaine lettuce, shallot, squash (butternut, spaghetti, acorn, etc.), sweet potatoes, tomatoes, yams, zucchini, etc. All vegetables are acceptable. Frozen vegetables are acceptable, especially when added to smoothies to add bulk and fiber, which reduces the speed sugar enters the blood.

FOODS TO LEAVE AT THE STORE

- Alcohol: beer, wine, spirits, and over-the-counter medicines/products that contain alcohol (mouthwash, cough syrups).
- Caffeine: caffeinated soda, coffee, energy drinks, guarana, tea, dark chocolate, coffee-flavored desserts, over-the-counter medications containing caffeine (Excedrin, etc.).
- Certain natural sugars: high-glycemic fruits (such as mango, pineapple, and watermelon), honey, maple syrup, brown, white or demerara sugar. Honestly, as long as you do not overeat, a small amount of sweet fruits is okay. You also have to be a bit gentle with yourself with sugar containing sauces like hoisin sauce. Does it contain sugar? Yes. Is it enough to kill your cleanse? No. As long as the sauce has less 2 or 3 g of sugar, you'll be okay.
- Chemical sugar substitutes: Equal, Splenda, Sweet'n Low, etc.
- Dairy: animal milk (cow, goat, camel, sheep, etc.), butter, cheese, cream, frozen yogurt, ice cream, sour cream, whipped cream, yogurt.
- Genetically modified anything: beet sugars, cane sugar, canola, corn, soy, etc.
- Gluten: bagels, bread, cake, cookies, couscous, crackers, deli meats, flour tortillas, muffins, pancakes, pasta, seitan, soy sauce, wheat flour, etc. Look for gluten-free cousins, but be sure you aren't accidentally including eggs.
- Meat and Eggs: beef, bison, cephalopods, chicken, duck, elk, fish, goat, lamb, mollusks, pork, quail, shellfish, squab, turkey, veal, venison, eggs, etc. If it had a mama, don't eat it.
- Processed Sugar: cakes, candy, cookies, fruit juice, pastries, soda, sorbet, condiments that contain sugar or high fructose corn syrup (HFCS) such as ketchup, steak sauce, etc.

SAMPLE MEAL PLAN

Nowhere is it set in stone that you must follow this meal plan. However, some people find it easier when there are instructions for what to eat each day. For those people, voilà, I present the meal plan. Honestly, unless you are cooking for a large family, you will likely not be able to eat all of the foods in this meal plan. However, you can look at the meal prep lists and pick which recipes you would like from those that are listed. If you don't like these recipes, no worries. Be creative, find your favorite recipe, and get cooking. Again, the most important thing is that you actually prepare food. This cleanse can be easy to dial in, with some people living on just carrot sticks and hummus for days. Don't do that. Cook meals and learn the joy of eating vegetables.

DAY 1
B: Chia Breakfast Pudding and Green Juice
L: Tofu, Mushroom and Bok Choy Bowls
D: Mediterranean Sweet Potatoes

DAY 2
B: Blueberry Bake
L: Mediterranean Chickpea Salad
D: Green Curry with Tofu and Peppers

DAY 3
B: Leftover Chia Pudding and Sunrise Turmeric Juice
L: Rice Salad
D: Lettuce Wraps

DAY 4
B: Leftover Blueberry Bake
L: Tofu and Mushroom Soup
D: Ratatouille

DAY 5
B: Mini-Frittata Muffins and Lemon-Lime Purple Cabbage Juice
L: Leftover Ratatouille
D: Wild Mushroom Soup

DAY 6

B: Southwest Tofu Scramble and Tomato Radish Juice

L: Caesar Salad

D: French Lentil and Potato Stew

DAY 7

B: Banana Porridge

L: Butternut Squash Soup

D: Trio of Sides: Roasted Brussels Sprouts with Grapes, Roasted Romanesco Broccoli, Grilled Lemon
   Garlic Zucchini

DAY 8

B: Steel Cut Oats

L: Vegan Egg Salad

D: Mushroom-Lentil Burgers and Sweet Potato Fries

DAY 9

B: Simple Chia Breakfast Bowl and Green Mint Lemonade

L: Sprouted Green Lentil Salad

D: Coconut Turmeric Spaghetti Squash Soup

DAY 10

B: Apple Crumble

L: Leftover Mushroom-Lentil Burgers

D: Coconut Curry Tempeh

DAY 11

B: Berry and Banana Porridge and Beet, Carrot, Ginger Juice

L: Caramelized Onion, Fig and Arugula Pizza

D: Leek, Apple, and Fennel Soup

DAY 12

B: Pumpkin Pancakes

L: Leftover Leek, Apple, and Fennel Soup

D: Quartet of Sides: Spinach Balls, Eggplant Mezze, Roasted Parmesan Chickpeas, Roasted Root
   Vegetable Medley

DAY 13

B: Latkes and Lavender Lemonade

L: Broccoli, Cheese and Rice Stuffed Peppers

D: Sushi Bowl

DAY 14

B: Enchilada Breakfast Casserole

L: Spaghetti with Fresh Marinara Sauce

D: Vietnamese Summer Rolls and Garlic Bok Choy

DAY 15

B: Leftover Enchilada Breakfast Casserole and Refreshing Romaine Lettuce Juice

L: Mac and Cheese

D: Borscht

DAY 16

B: Cauliflower Hash Browns

L: Butternut Squash and Lemon Quinoa

D: Jackfruit Tacos and Mexican Pinto Bean Salad

DAY 17

B: Pumpkin Chia Pudding and Spicy Cucumber Cooler

L: Cauliflower Steaks with Parsnip Purée and Lemon-Caper Sauce

D: Collard Green Wraps

DAY 18

B: Peach and Berry Crisp

L: Mexican Burrito Bowl

D: Vietnamese Cauliflower Soup with Roasted Cauliflower

DAY 19

B: Steel Cut Oats with Caramelized Bananas and Virgin Mary

L: Tomato and Cucumber Salad

D: Broccoli and Cheese Muffins and Spinach Salad

DAY 20

B: Sweet Potato and Kale Hash

L: Broccoli Salad

D: Hearty Potato Soup

DAY 21

B: Tomato Basil Chickpea Omelets and Cranberry Soda

L: Your New Dish

D: Buffalo Cauliflower Tacos and Banana Ice Cream

WEEKLY FOOD PREP

1. Prepare your breakfast for Day 1: Simple Chia Bowl.
2. For Day 1 lunch, the entire recipe can be made in advance and reheated.
3. For Day 1 dinner, bake sweet potatoes, and make hummus.
4. For Day 2 breakfast, you can make the entire recipe and wrap for on-the-go options.
5. For Day 3 lunch, you may want to shred carrots or radishes in advance.
6. For Day 6 lunch, make salad dressing and store in refrigerator.
7. For Day 7 dinner, cut broccoli and cauliflower.
8. Cut carrots, celery, zucchini and other fresh vegetables for snacks throughout the week.
9. Make vegan mayonnaise (see recipes in the *CSC Cookbook* p.38 – 40) for easy wraps and sandwiches through the week.
10. Make vegetable stock (see recipe in the *CSC Cookbook* p. 42) for use through the week.

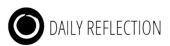 DAILY REFLECTION

Take time to think about why you are going to do this cleanse. Cleansing isn't difficult, but it does require you to commit to doing it. You need to dedicate time to planning meals, grocery shopping and cooking.

Think about how you want to feel at the end of the 21 days. Give your body a clean slate and let's crush it!

You got this.

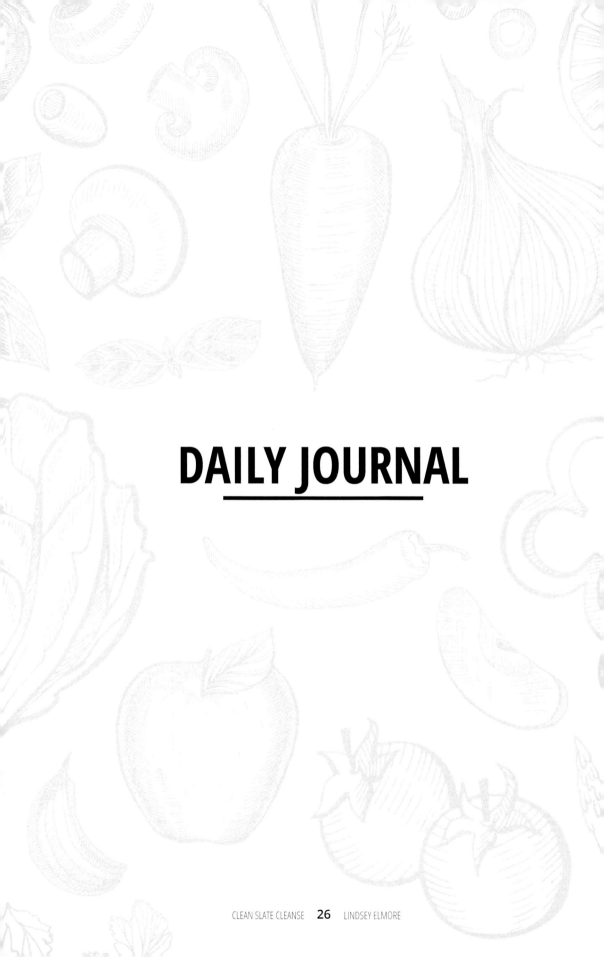

DAILY JOURNAL

INACTION BREEDS
DOUBT & FEAR.

action

BREEDS CONFIDENCE
AND COURAGE

- DALE CARNEGIE -

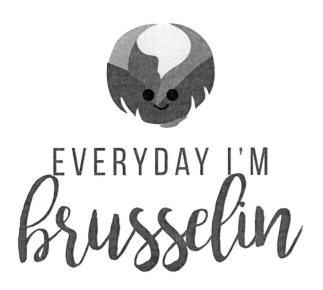

EVERYDAY I'M
brusselin

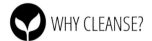 # WHY CLEANSE?

Starting on a cleanse is not the easiest thing in the world to do. It takes dedication, persistence, and planning. You first have to admit that you need a change to your routine, and then be brave enough to actually change. But when you go for it and achieve the goal of sticking to this plan for a full 3 weeks, you will experience a lot of positive changes.

When you stick to the cleanse, the changes in your body and mind can far exceed the initial struggle and perceived sacrifice. For example, plant-based cleanses can provide many health benefits, and these are summarized here:

HEALTH BENEFITS OF VEGAN AND VEGETARIAN CLEANSES:
1. Decreased body weight[1,2]
2. Decreased waist and hip circumference[2]
3. Decreased blood pressure[2,3]
4. Decrease in total cholesterol and low-density lipoprotein (LDL, 'bad') cholesterol[1,2]
5. Reduced risk of coronary heart disease[4]
6. Reduced risk of diabetes and metabolic syndrome[4]
7. Increased testosterone in men[2]

While the effects on the mind are more difficult to quantify with data, I believe that cleanses can help renew our relationship with food. This cleanse includes a lot of mindful eating practices, meditations, and grounding exercises to help you through this process. Participants have expressed increased self-awareness, mental clarity, and mindfulness selecting foods. Cleansing and fasting has also been a part of many cultural and spiritual traditions in both Eastern and Western models of religion and spirituality.

Other less tangible effects include larger and more well-formed bowel movements (aka #pooptopia), as well as fresher breath, clearer skin, more energy, and increased sexual desire.

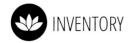 INVENTORY

For today's exercise, we will take inventory of why you decided to do the cleanse. This document will be great for you to look back on if it seems like there is no way you can survive another day. Remembering why you began will remind you of the confidence you have at this very moment, and what positive changes you hoped to see during the cleanse.

You will also craft your own positive affirmation to help remind you of how strong you are. I want you to create a statement in the present tense, and usually start with "I am. . ." Examples of statements include "I am living my healthiest life." Or "I have a healthy relationship with sugar and food." If you are struggling with underlying disease issues or food allergies, perhaps you can remind yourself that "I am able to digest all healthy food with grace and ease." There are some other statements that do not start with "I am. . . " such as "Every cell in my body is happy and healthy." Create as many of these statements as you like. These will be a great source of comfort and strength when you might be struggling. Take some time to think about the following questions and statements on the next page as you write out your affirmations.

1. Three reasons I decided to do this cleanse.

_____

_____

_____

2. What is the best thing that can happen when I succeed with this cleanse?

_____

3. What do I hope to accomplish in the next 21 days?

_____

4. What do I most look forward to?

_____

5. What challenges do I anticipate?

_____

_____

6. What will I do when challenges arise?

_____

7. Three new foods I am most excited to try.

_____

8. Three questions I have about this cleanse that I would like to research.

_____

_____

_____

9. In the next 21 days, what do I most want to see?

_____

10. At the end of this 21-day cleanse, I will be. . .

_____

11. What are 3 goals you hope to achieve? (This can be either during the cleanse or long term).

_____

_____

_____

12. Of these three goals, which is the most important to you?

_____

13. My affirmation statement.

_____

_____

_____

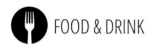

FOOD & DRINK

TODAY'S MENU

B: _____

L: _____

D: _____

REFLECTION ON THE DAY

HOW WAS YOUR SLEEP LAST NIGHT?

The worst, I barely slept   Like a rock

| 1 | 2 | 3 | 4 | 5 | 6 | 7 | 8 | 9 | 10 |

HOW IS YOUR ENERGY TODAY?

I am literally walking dead over here   I could probably run a marathon

| 1 | 2 | 3 | 4 | 5 | 6 | 7 | 8 | 9 | 10 |

THE QUALITY OF YOUR POOP THIS MORNING?

Smelly, severe constipation or diarrhea   Smooth, 10-12 inch masterpiece

| 1 | 2 | 3 | 4 | 5 | 6 | 7 | 8 | 9 | 10 |

HOW ARE YOUR FOOD CRAVINGS TODAY?

Somebody give me a doughnut now   What's to crave? This food is amazing!

| 1 | 2 | 3 | 4 | 5 | 6 | 7 | 8 | 9 | 10 |

REFLECTION ON TODAY

_____

_____

☐ CRUSHED IT!

THE PESSIMIST SEES DIFFICULTY
IN EVERY OPPORTUNITY.

THE OPTIMIST SEES
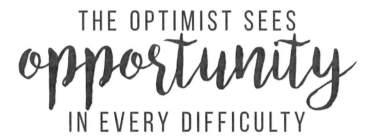
IN EVERY DIFFICULTY

- WINSTON CHURCHILL -

CAFFEINE MAY:

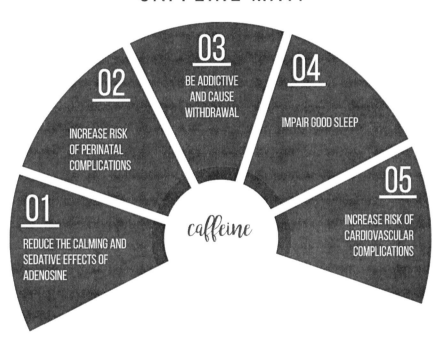

02 INCREASE RISK OF PERINATAL COMPLICATIONS

03 BE ADDICTIVE AND CAUSE WITHDRAWAL

04 IMPAIR GOOD SLEEP

01 REDUCE THE CALMING AND SEDATIVE EFFECTS OF ADENOSINE

05 INCREASE RISK OF CARDIOVASCULAR COMPLICATIONS

caffeine

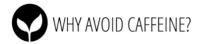# WHY AVOID CAFFEINE?

For many people, giving up caffeine is one of the most difficult parts of this cleanse. Morning routines can be defined with coffee or tea, a newspaper, a podcast or a news program on television. Caffeine is the most commonly used drug in the world, and it is used by 90% of adults in the United States.[1] Caffeine is found in coffee, tea, and chocolate and is an additive in sodas, candies, and energy shots. Among Americans who use caffeine, the average consumption is approximately 200 mg/day.[2]

But it brings with it a broad array of potential risks. Caffeine increases the risk of cardiovascular complications (such as increased blood pressure, arrhythmias, increased heart rate, and even more serious complications such as heart attack, and death) and perinatal complications (such as low birth weight).[3-7]

Caffeine binds and antagonizes (blocks the effects of) the adenosine receptor, and this leads to a variety of effects opposite to the effects of adenosine. Adenosine is a natural hormone that promotes sleep and suppresses arousal, increases the diameter of blood vessels and has an anti-platelet action, thus increasing blood flow and increasing relaxation.[8] When the effects of adenosine are blocked by caffeine, it leads to short-term alertness and stimulant effects. Caffeine also binds to dopamine receptors and prevents adenosine's down-regulatory influence at dopamine receptors. Engagement of the dopamine receptor may be the underlying cause of the addictive potential of caffeine, especially since caffeine engages dopamine receptors in the same area of the brain as amphetamines and cocaine.[9-11]

Through a complex system, caffeine increases the amount of adrenaline in the body. Inside the cell, caffeine blocks the breakdown of cyclic-adenosine monophosphate (cAMP), and its effects are prolonged and amplified. In the heart, this prompts adrenaline and nor-adrenaline to increase the rate and force of muscle contraction.[12-14] In the rest of the body, the 'fight or flight' behavior mechanisms are engaged.[15] There is also evidence that caffeine can work directly on adrenal cells to mobilize calcium and increase the excretion of both adrenaline and nor-adrenaline directly from mammalian adrenal cells.[16]

Caffeine stays in the body for about 4 to 5 hours after ingestion and stays much longer in infants and young children (up to 100 hrs.) and in women who are pregnant. Caffeine must be metabolized by the liver before it is prepared for excretion, and therefore it taxes the liver. Caffeine is cleared more slowly from the body if there is liver damage.[17]

The great news is that there are plenty of alternatives to caffeinated beverages. Pick your favorite and give it a go today. Here are a few of my favorites:

1. Warm lemon water first thing in the morning.
2. Peppermint tea for the morning.
3. Ginger or lemon tea after a meal.
4. Chamomile tea in the evening.
5. Energizing essential oils such as rosemary, cinnamon, peppermint, and lemongrass.
6. Club soda-based mocktails.

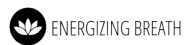 ## ENERGIZING BREATH

Grab some peppermint essential oil. (If you don't have peppermint essential oil, grab some peppermint leaves, and tear them in your hands. And by the way, you totally need some essential oils.)

1. Cup your hand over your mouth and nose and gently inhale the peppermint aroma. Exhale. Inhale. Exhale. Inhale. Exhale.
2. Come to a standing position with your feet hip-distance apart. Gently bend your knees. Take a big inhale as you gently lift your arms over your head. Exhale as you lower your arms. Repeat: inhale as you lift your arms over your head. Exhale as you lower. And one last time: inhale as you lift your arms over your head. Exhale as you lower.
3. Bring your hands over your mouth again. Say your affirmation from yesterday aloud three times. Inhale and exhale for three breaths while inhaling the scent of peppermint. Say your affirmation three times again. Finish with one more cycle of breaths.

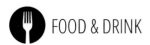 FOOD & DRINK

TODAY'S MENU

B: _____

L: _____

D: _____

REFLECTION ON THE DAY

HOW WAS YOUR SLEEP LAST NIGHT?

The worst, I barely slept   Like a rock

1   2   3   4   5   6   7   8   9   10

HOW IS YOUR ENERGY TODAY?

I am literally walking dead over here   I could probably run a marathon

1   2   3   4   5   6   7   8   9   10

THE QUALITY OF YOUR POOP THIS MORNING?

Smelly, severe constipation or diarrhea   Smooth, 10-12 inch masterpiece

1   2   3   4   5   6   7   8   9   10

HOW ARE YOUR FOOD CRAVINGS TODAY?

Somebody give me a doughnut now   What's to crave? This food is amazing!

1   2   3   4   5   6   7   8   9   10

REFLECTION ON TODAY

_____

_____

☐ CRUSHED IT!

FAILURE WILL NEVER
OVERTAKE ME IF MY

determination

TO SUCCEED IS STRONG ENOUGH

- O G   M A N D I N O -

PROCESSED SUGAR MAY:

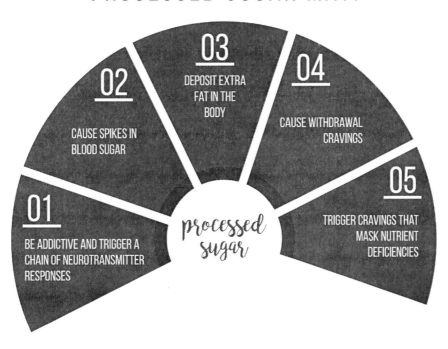

02 CAUSE SPIKES IN BLOOD SUGAR

03 DEPOSIT EXTRA FAT IN THE BODY

04 CAUSE WITHDRAWAL CRAVINGS

01 BE ADDICTIVE AND TRIGGER A CHAIN OF NEUROTRANSMITTER RESPONSES

05 TRIGGER CRAVINGS THAT MASK NUTRIENT DEFICIENCIES

processed sugar

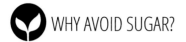 WHY AVOID SUGAR?

There are a wide variety of events that take place when the body is exposed to sugar. First, sugar triggers an addictive response in your brain very similar to drugs like heroin and cocaine. There are dramatic changes in neurotransmitters. Serotonin is increased, and this can lead to mood swings and changes in perception. Dopamine is increased, and this may lead to sugar dependence. The pain numbing opioid receptor is engaged, and feel good peptides known as enkephalins are released.[1]

Neurotransmitter imbalance is worsened because many sweet foods are used as rewards for good behavior, for celebrations, and for positive affirmations. We learn to associate sugar with reward, and the addictive cycle continues. Some authors contend that sugar is even more addictive than drugs of abuse.[2]

Sugar may also be addictive because of how it impacts insulin. When blood sugar levels spike, massive amounts of insulin are secreted. The surge of insulin then causes blood sugar to fall rapidly, and this causes immediate storage of fat in the tissues. As the liver converts sugar into fat and deposits it in the body, blood sugar levels rapidly plummet, and this causes additional cravings to restore the high that was lost.

Sugar cravings may signal a lot of bad things at work in your body. They can be a strong indicator of insulin resistance or signal that you are deficient in nutrients or water. Consumption of a diet high in sugar-laden, unhealthy food can trigger mineral deficiencies, creating a cycle of cravings that do nothing to solve the underlying nutrient deficiency.[3]

Sugar contributes to the growth of candida in the body. This fungus can cause infections, gas, irritable bowel syndrome, and fluid retention, as well as fatigue and anxiety. It is sometimes said that sugar feeds cancer, and that is because when we eat sugar, the body releases insulin to bring the sugar levels down. The more insulin that you have in your body, the more cancer cells can proliferate.

Artificial sugars are no better and may actually be worse for you. So many people use artificial sugars such as aspartame, sucralose, and saccharin thinking that they will reduce the risk of adverse effects like diabetes, weight gain, and cardiovascular disease. But a growing body of evidence indicates that the risk is actually higher with artificial sweeteners versus natural sweeteners.[4] Also, since artificial sweeteners are more than 1,000 times more potent than regular sugars, they alter your palate requiring that you eat more to get the same effect.

OVERCOMING TEMPTATION WITH ACTIONABLE PLANS

What will you do when challenges arise? Here are a couple of ideas:

Create positive affirmations that will help you overcome challenges. Back when I was coaching others on quitting smoking, I found some of their positive statements extraordinarily inspiring. For example, one of my patients would often remind herself, "Just because I am thinking about a cigarette doesn't mean I have to have one." Another patient told himself, "I love myself more than I love a cigarette." You can use statements like these for food as well. "Just because I am thinking about pizza doesn't mean I have to eat it."

Create alternative solutions to eating unhealthy foods. When chocolate cake seems to be calling your name, what are 3 positive activities that may help you stay on course for your goals? Consider a 5-minute walk, 7 deep breaths, going to a movie or play, calling a friend, writing in your journal, playing a game with your kids, or doing 3 sun salutations. There are so many easy activities that can distract your mind away from the food in front of you. Find something that inspires you and know that you have it as a fall back plan when times get tough.

1. List three ways that you will prepare for difficult times you will face in the next 3 weeks.

_____

_____

_____

2. What are 3 alternative solutions to eating unhealthy foods?

_____

_____

_____

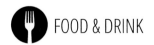 FOOD & DRINK

TODAY'S MENU

B: _____

L: _____

D: _____

REFLECTION ON THE DAY

HOW WAS YOUR SLEEP LAST NIGHT?

The worst, I barely slept   Like a rock

1   2   3   4   5   6   7   8   9   10

HOW IS YOUR ENERGY TODAY?

I am literally walking dead over here   I could probably run a marathon

1   2   3   4   5   6   7   8   9   10

THE QUALITY OF YOUR POOP THIS MORNING?

Smelly, severe constipation or diarrhea   Smooth, 10-12 inch masterpiece

1   2   3   4   5   6   7   8   9   10

HOW ARE YOUR FOOD CRAVINGS TODAY?

Somebody give me a doughnut now   What's to crave? This food is amazing!

1   2   3   4   5   6   7   8   9   10

REFLECTION ON TODAY

_____

_____

☐ CRUSHED IT!

NO ONE IS BORN A

great cook

ONE LEARNS BY DOING.

- JULIA CHILD -

MEAT & DAIRY PRODUCTS MAY:

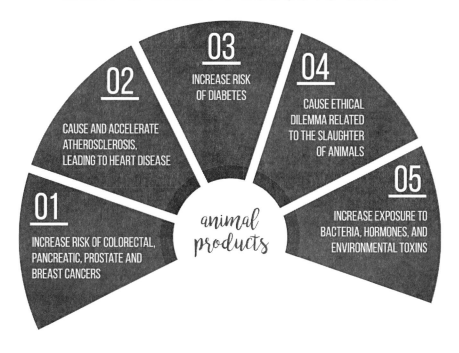

01 INCREASE RISK OF COLORECTAL, PANCREATIC, PROSTATE AND BREAST CANCERS

02 CAUSE AND ACCELERATE ATHEROSCLEROSIS, LEADING TO HEART DISEASE

03 INCREASE RISK OF DIABETES

04 CAUSE ETHICAL DILEMMA RELATED TO THE SLAUGHTER OF ANIMALS

05 INCREASE EXPOSURE TO BACTERIA, HORMONES, AND ENVIRONMENTAL TOXINS

animal products

WHY AVOID MEAT AND ANIMAL PRODUCTS?

Perhaps the most controversial part of this cleanse is the exclusion of meat and animal products. Some people feel passionately that humans need meat to survive and thrive, where others feel equally as passionately against the notion. This cleanse is not intended to necessarily sway you to eat plant-based for life, but it is intended to make you think about the animal products that you choose to bring into your body.

The joint opinion of the American Dietetic Association and Dieticians of Canada is that vegetarian lifestyles are safe for people of all ages, races, and genders.[1] Some contend that you must receive critical nutrition such as Vitamin B12, protein, and omega-3 fatty acids from meat, but I contend that humans can live healthy vibrant lives without consumption of any animal products. For more on this discussion, please see Day 10 reading on Common Questions on Plant Based Diets.

For Day 4 and Day 14, let's take a look at the data related to potential harm from consumption of meat and other animal products.

ANIMAL PRODUCTS AND CANCER

After reviewing more than 800 studies across many different countries, the World Health Organization lists processed meats and salted fish as class 1 carcinogens known to cause cancer in humans (same as asbestos, cigarette smoking, and plutonium). Processed meat includes any meat that has been transformed through salting, curing, fermenting, smoking or other process to improve preservation. This includes hot dogs, ham, sausages, corned beef, beef jerky, canned meats and meat-based preparations and sauces. This classification was made based on sufficient evidence to conclude that consumption of processed meat causes colorectal cancer, and the expert panel concluded that each 50g portion of processed meat eaten daily increases the risk of colorectal cancer by 18%.[2]

All red meats are classified as a class 2A carcinogen (same as lead, mustard gas, DDT), and are probably cancer-causing in humans. Red meat is defined as any mammalian muscle meat: beef, pork, veal, lamb, goat, horse, or mutton. The conclusion was made based on limited evidence that consumption of these products is related to colorectal cancer, pancreatic cancer, and prostate cancer with strong mechanistic evidence of how meat supports the formation of cancers.[2]

The typical Western diet (comprised of high intake of fatty and sugary foods as well as red meat) has been shown in case control studies to increase the risk of breast cancer in pre- and post-menopausal women by 68% and 48%, respectively.[3]

Casein is a combination of proteins contained in dairy products including milk, yogurt, kefir cheese, and ice cream. α-Casein and combined caseins have both been shown to promote the growth of certain strains of prostate cancer cells in vitro. This relationship is dose dependent, so the greater the exposure to casein, the larger the cancer cell growth. Casein concentration is 10 times higher in cow's milk than human milk.[4]

ANIMAL PRODUCTS AND HEART DISEASE

There is good evidence to suggest that animal products increase the risk of atherosclerosis (the buildup of fats, cholesterol, and other substances in the artery walls), and that transitioning to a plant-based diet reduces cholesterol an average of 35%.[5,6]

We now know that meat and animal product consumption can accelerate atherosclerosis as well. The acceleration may be because meat consumption changes the bacteria in the gut and drives the gut to favor bacteria more likely to produce trimethylamine oxide (TMAO).[5] When we eat a diet that is high in meat, we eat a diet high in carnitine and choline. Since we have lots of carnitine in our guts, we recruit bacteria that metabolize carnitine and choline. Gut bacteria convert carnitine to trimethylamine, and then the liver converts it to TMAO. TMAO then reduces the absorption of cholesterol in arteries and accelerates atherosclerotic plaque growth. In the same article, fasting plasma carnitine levels were linked to the risk of major cardiac events including death, heart attack, stroke, and revascularization. It was found that high levels of carnitine increased the risk for one of these events, and that it was directly linked to the gut bacteria and the production of pro-inflammatory TMAO.

Amazingly, replacing just 1% of energy from animal protein with plant protein has been associated with an 18% reduction in the risk of developing type 2 diabetes. And on the flip side, replacing 1% of carbohydrate energy from plants with energy from protein increased the risk of developing type 2 diabetes by 5%.[7]

There is controversy about whether or not eggs can lead to or worsen diabetes. In one study, people who eat more than 1 egg per day are 42% more likely to get diabetes, and in people who already have diabetes, consumption of more than 1 egg per day increases the risk of a cardiac event by 69%.[8] However, the risk of eating eggs and developing diabetes is not universally duplicated in studies.[7] In another study, higher egg consumption was associated with higher blood sugar in people with diabetes or impaired fasting glucose.[9]

It is known that milk, and the casein proteins contained within, increase insulin and insulin-like growth factor, and this leads to growth in pre-pubertal boys.[10] The effects are only from dairy, not meat.[11] We have also seen in other studies that higher levels of carnitine in the blood have been associated with an increased risk of heart attack, stroke, and death in people undergoing cardiac evaluations.

SUMMARY

As we can see from the selection of evidence above, there are a wide variety of reasons to avoid meat and animal products for at least a short period of time. There are also a wide variety of health benefits, including a decreased risk of cardiovascular disease and cancer, associated with removing meat from the diet. There are also many environmental benefits that come from reducing meat consumption, and these points will be covered in a later chapter.

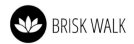 BRISK WALK

The sugar and caffeine crash can be really tough in the first few days on a cleanse. Instead of reaching for the foods that we are so used to, let's shift our perspective and go outside for a brisk walk. Taking a brisk walk can help you maintain a healthy weight, prevent high blood pressure, diabetes, and other cardiovascular disease, strengthen your bones and muscles, improve mood, and improve balance and coordination. Don't feel the need to be a champion. If you have led a sedentary lifestyle for an extended period of time, simply taking 15 minutes to go outside, breathing in the fresh air and soaking up the sunshine can be a simple way to facilitate detoxification through breath and maybe even a bit of sweat.

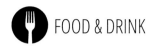 FOOD & DRINK

TODAY'S MENU

B: _____

L: _____

D: _____

REFLECTION ON THE DAY

HOW WAS YOUR SLEEP LAST NIGHT?

The worst, I barely slept   Like a rock

1   2   3   4   5   6   7   8   9   10

HOW IS YOUR ENERGY TODAY?

I am literally walking dead over here   I could probably run a marathon

1   2   3   4   5   6   7   8   9   10

THE QUALITY OF YOUR POOP THIS MORNING?

Smelly, severe constipation or diarrhea   Smooth, 10-12 inch masterpiece

1   2   3   4   5   6   7   8   9   10

HOW ARE YOUR FOOD CRAVINGS TODAY?

Somebody give me a doughnut now   What's to crave? This food is amazing!

1   2   3   4   5   6   7   8   9   10

REFLECTION ON TODAY

_____

_____

☐ CRUSHED IT!

GOD GRANT ME THE
SERENITY TO ACCEPT
THINGS I CANNOT CHANGE,
THE COURAGE TO
CHANGE THE THINGS I CAN,
**AND THE WISDOM TO
KNOW THE DIFFERENCE.**

- ALCOHOLICS ANONYMOUS
SERENITY PRAYERR -

ALCOHOL MAY:

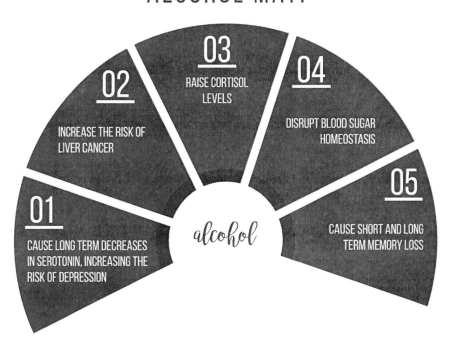

01 CAUSE LONG TERM DECREASES IN SEROTONIN, INCREASING THE RISK OF DEPRESSION

02 INCREASE THE RISK OF LIVER CANCER

03 RAISE CORTISOL LEVELS

04 DISRUPT BLOOD SUGAR HOMEOSTASIS

05 CAUSE SHORT AND LONG TERM MEMORY LOSS

alcohol

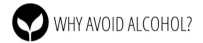 WHY AVOID ALCOHOL?

EFFECTS ON THE BRAIN

Alcohol interferes with GABA, serotonin, and dopamine. One drink temporarily increases serotonin, which elevates mood and thinking. However, over time, alcohol can lower serotonin levels, causing mood swings and depression. It also interacts with tryptophan (a natural mood elevator). Alcohol increases the amount of GABA and this slows down the brain input. This is what leads to the look of someone who has had a few drinks. It also increases dopamine, which reinforces feelings of reward. The body handles alcohol like a toxin, and therefore it must be processed via the liver, and this fatigues the liver.

EFFECTS ON BLOOD SUGAR AND HORMONES

There are strange effects on blood sugar: alcohol decreases blood sugar, but the sugar that we take in with it increases blood sugar. The pancreas releases insulin, which decreases blood sugar. The liver is using energy to detoxify alcohol instead of building sugar storage molecules (glycogen). This is why it is easier to give up alcohol and sugar at the same time.

Alcohol raises cortisol levels, and this can further destabilize blood sugars. It depletes vitamins, especially B vitamins, and these are critical for a normal stress response. Lastly, alcohol inhibits our ability to get REM sleep, and this means that you don't wake as rested as you could have without alcohol.

CARDIOVASCULAR EFFECTS

Though low-to-moderate amounts of alcohol intake are associated with improvements in cardiovascular health, ethanol chronically consumed in large amounts is a toxin to the heart and vasculature. Long-term heavy use of alcohol can produce cardiac injury and progress to heart failure and eventual death.[1]

CARCINOGENICITY

Lastly, the World Health Organization lists alcohol as a class 1 carcinogen, and it may be associated with head and neck,[2] esophageal,[3] liver,[4] breast,[5] and colorectal cancers.[6] This is because the breakdown of alcohol leads to the production of acetaldehyde, and this is known to disrupt DNA. Alcohol also generates free oxygen species, and impairs the body's ability to absorb and break down a variety of nutrients, including vitamins A, B9, B12, C, D, E and carotenoids. Alcohol increases estrogens, which can increase the occurrence of breast cancers.[7]

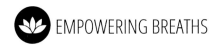 EMPOWERING BREATHS

When I was living in San Francisco, I learned a lot about food and beverage culture, and I learned to love it. I love a good glass of wine or a cocktail with a fancy schmancy dinner. When I am cleansing, or simply don't feel like drinking, I love to use this empowering breathing exercise before I head out to dinner with friends and family whom I know will be drinking. This is called the "Ha!" breath exercise, and you have to really make some noise to get the full benefits! Really pay attention to the way the shape of your belly changes as you breathe in and out. This makes a big difference.

HA! BREATH EXERCISE

1. For this exercise, grab a bottle of lemon oil and add a few drops to your hands. If you don't have lemon essential oil, you can smell lemon peels or lemon zest.
2. Bring your feet hip distance apart and bend your knees a bit. Place your hands over your mouth and nose and gently inhale and exhale for three breaths.
3. Lower your hands and bring them to rest on your solar plexus. This is the space between your ribs above your belly button.
4. Take a deep breath in and allow your belly to distend, and as you exhale allow your belly to pull back in toward your spine.
5. Now we are going to do this with a bit more force.
6. Take a quick inhale of your lemon aroma.
7. Place your hands back on your solar plexus. Take a deep inhale and allow your belly to distend. As you exhale, give a loud and audible "Ha!" as you quickly bring your navel back toward your spine.
8. Do this again, and really open your mouth and let out an audible "Ha!"

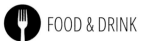 FOOD & DRINK

TODAY'S MENU

B: _____

L: _____

D: _____

REFLECTION ON THE DAY

HOW WAS YOUR SLEEP LAST NIGHT?

The worst, I barely slept   Like a rock

1   2   3   4   5   6   7   8   9   10

HOW IS YOUR ENERGY TODAY?

I am literally walking dead over here   I could probably run a marathon

1   2   3   4   5   6   7   8   9   10

THE QUALITY OF YOUR POOP THIS MORNING?

Smelly, severe constipation or diarrhea   Smooth, 10-12 inch masterpiece

1   2   3   4   5   6   7   8   9   10

HOW ARE YOUR FOOD CRAVINGS TODAY?

Somebody give me a doughnut now   What's to crave? This food is amazing!

1   2   3   4   5   6   7   8   9   10

REFLECTION ON TODAY

_____

_____

☐ CRUSHED IT!

THE
only limit
TO OUR REALIZATION OF
TOMORROW WILL BE OUR
DOUBTS OF TODAY

- FRANKLIN D. ROOSEVELT -

GLUTEN MAY:

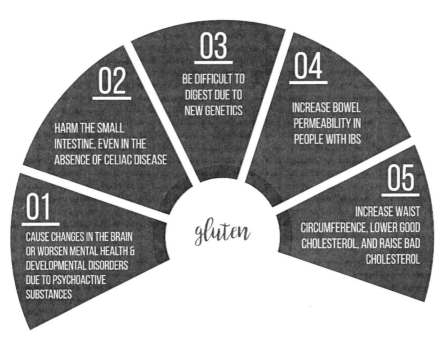

02 HARM THE SMALL INTESTINE, EVEN IN THE ABSENCE OF CELIAC DISEASE

03 BE DIFFICULT TO DIGEST DUE TO NEW GENETICS

04 INCREASE BOWEL PERMEABILITY IN PEOPLE WITH IBS

01 CAUSE CHANGES IN THE BRAIN OR WORSEN MENTAL HEALTH & DEVELOPMENTAL DISORDERS DUE TO PSYCHOACTIVE SUBSTANCES

05 INCREASE WAIST CIRCUMFERENCE, LOWER GOOD CHOLESTEROL, AND RAISE BAD CHOLESTEROL

gluten

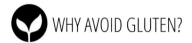# WHY AVOID GLUTEN?

Wheat has been through a dramatic transformation in the past 200 years, and some contend that it has created an epidemic of allergies and sensitivities to gluten. Gluten is a stretchy protein that acts like a glue and maintains the shape and texture of breads.

One of the most ancient forms of wheat is called Einkorn, and its genetic code is dramatically different than modern wheat. Einkorn has 14 chromosomes, while modern wheat has 42. Einkorn contains only the A genome of wheat. Modern wheat, on the other hand, has been crossed with 2 goat grasses. This introduced the D genome, and it makes up about 5% of the entire genetic code. Bakers love the D genome, because the glutens in this family bounce back quicker and provide a quick, high rise. But it has also introduced new genetics to the flours, and this may make modern wheat more difficult to digest.[1]

There is some research that suggests gluten harms the small intestine, and the damage allows food peptides to be released into the body, even in the absence of celiac disease. When this happens, the body goes into overdrive and creates an over blown immune response. They damage the villi in the gut, which inhibits our body's ability to absorb nutrients. The effects of gluten can be subtle: headaches, asthma, skin rashes, weight gain, bloating, all the way to celiac disease.

Celiac disease is a serious autoimmune disease whereby gluten leads to major damage in the small intestine.[2] Though only 1-2% of the United States population is diagnosed with celiac disease, there is some evidence to suggest that up to 80% of people with celiac disease are unaware,[3] and that non-celiac gluten sensitivity is much more common.

In people with irritable bowel syndrome where diarrhea (IBS-D) is the prominent symptom, gluten increases the permeability of the small bowel and alters bowel barrier function.[4] Eliminating gluten as a part of the low FODMAP diet (Fermentable Oligo-, Di-, Mono-saccharides And Polyols), can improve the individual symptoms of irritable bowel syndrome, particularly pain and bloating.[5]

The food peptides in gluten have a major impact on the brain. It contains a neuro-active peptide called gliadorphin-7, one of many different exorphins. Other exorphins include casein from dairy, soymorphins from soy, and rubiscolins from spinach. Exorphins bind the opioid receptor, the same receptor in the brain to which pain killers bind. Not only can dietary exorphins create abnormal behaviors in rodents, there is evidence to suggest that removing gluten from the diet can relieve abnormal behaviors in people with schizophrenia. Furthermore, removing gluten and casein from the diet can improve behavior in 81%

of children with autism.[6,7] There have been case reports of dramatic turnarounds following at least 3 months without gluten and dairy.

There is evidence to suggest that in people without celiac disease, those who avoid gluten are more likely to have a smaller waist circumference, higher high-density lipoprotein (HDL) cholesterol, and higher self-reported weight loss over the course of one year. There was also a decrease in the probability of having metabolic syndrome and lower 10-year CVD risk scores.[8]

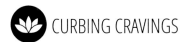# CURBING CRAVINGS

Bread can be one of the most craveable foods out there. There is something so comforting about the smell of fresh baked bread, the crunch of the crust, and the way that butter melts into it or olive oil is absorbed. Certainly no one is denying that it is delicious, but as we have just learned, it can be inflammatory and brain changing. I adapted today's exercise from the *Meditation Minis Podcast* by Chel Hamilton.[9] I love this podcast because they are all really short meditations, and there are many to choose from.

1. Grab a bottle of ocotea essential oil (or the essential oil of your choice) and inhale the scent from the bottle for three breaths. Let out a sigh on the exhale, as you give your body permission to relax.
2. Come to a comfortable seated position. If you are in a chair, bring your feet flat on the floor and your hands gently resting on your lap.
3. As it is comfortable, invite your eyes to close.
4. I want you to envision a luxurious bread basket right in front of you. Warm from the oven, smelling indulgent. There are many different kinds of breads to choose from: crusty baguettes, soft dinner rolls, oily focaccia, and chewy ciabatta. There are also spreads of your choice: olive oil, vinegar, butter, pesto, you name it.
5. Take inventory of your body now. On a scale of 1-10 how strong is your craving for the food? With 1 being, "eh, I don't even care" to 10 being, "must have bread!" Where do you sense that craving in your body? Does it have a shape or a form? Maybe you see it as a color. Or just as a general sense.
6. As quickly as the craving for the bread or any other food arises, I want you to imagine brushing it off of the table as you would bread crumbs. Just a swift little flick of the wrist brushes away the craving so that it no longer affects you. Maybe you find that there are a lot of crumbs to brush away. That's okay. They are lightweight, and easily under your control to move away from you.
7. Maybe as you are brushing away the breadcrumbs, another craving pops into your mind. That's okay. It can be brushed away like breadcrumbs too. Whatever the food is, gently see it moving off the side of the table.
8. Take three additional breaths, inhaling your essential oil from the bottle.

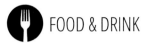 FOOD & DRINK

TODAY'S MENU

B: _____

L: _____

D: _____

REFLECTION ON THE DAY

HOW WAS YOUR SLEEP LAST NIGHT?

The worst, I barely slept   Like a rock

| 1 | 2 | 3 | 4 | 5 | 6 | 7 | 8 | 9 | 10 |

HOW IS YOUR ENERGY TODAY?

I am literally walking dead over here   I could probably run a marathon

| 1 | 2 | 3 | 4 | 5 | 6 | 7 | 8 | 9 | 10 |

THE QUALITY OF YOUR POOP THIS MORNING?

Smelly, severe constipation or diarrhea   Smooth, 10-12 inch masterpiece

| 1 | 2 | 3 | 4 | 5 | 6 | 7 | 8 | 9 | 10 |

HOW ARE YOUR FOOD CRAVINGS TODAY?

Somebody give me a doughnut now   What's to crave? This food is amazing!

| 1 | 2 | 3 | 4 | 5 | 6 | 7 | 8 | 9 | 10 |

REFLECTION ON TODAY

_____

_____

☐ CRUSHED IT!

SLEEP IS THE BEST

meditation

- DALAI LAMA -

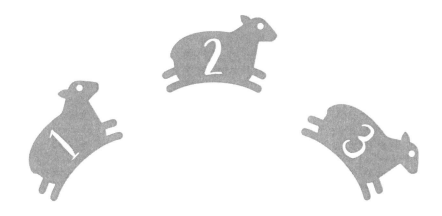

THE IMPORTANCE OF WATER AND SLEEP

Our bodies are comprised of approximately 50-75% water, making it the most abundant molecule in the body, and almost each body system is dependent on it to function properly. Death may result in as little as 2-3 days without water, whereas humans can survive for months without food. Water is required to maintain homeostasis and has a long list of benefits to human health.

The brain is very highly dependent on water for optimal functioning, and a wide variety of studies have shown that dehydration can affect mood, memory, and brain performance in children, adults and the elderly.[1-3] Even mild dehydration can affect mood in young women. In this same study, dehydrated women perceived tasks as more challenging, had reduced levels of concentration, and complained of headaches.[4] Dehydration is a common cause of both tension-type headache and migraine headache.[5] In people who are dehydrated, water can cure the symptoms of certain types of headache. At a minimum, it may reduce the intensity and duration.[6]

During exercise, water helps to maximize physical and mental performance. When dehydrated, exercise feels more challenging, motivation is reduced, and body temperatures are harder to regulate.[7] Adequate hydration may reduce oxidative stress that occurs during high intensity exercise.[8]

Water also has an impact on metabolism, waste excretion, and cravings. Water can also increase thermogenesis and aid in weight loss. When inadequately hydrated, we may suffer from food cravings, especially sugar cravings. When our bowels are adequately moving, we also have a greater ability to eliminate toxins and wastes from our bodies, and water helps to lubricate the bowels and reduce symptoms of constipation.[9]

Sleep is critically important to our health, body weight and hormone function. People who do not get enough sleep tend to have heavier body weights and increased body mass index. In a meta-analysis of more than 640,000 children and adults, it was found that children who do not get adequate sleep were 89% more likely to be obese and adults were 55% more likely to be obese. Lack of sleep is associated with increase caloric intake, altered hormone function, and poor appetite regulation.[10] Specifically, there is a reduction in the amount of leptin (a hormone that suppresses appetite) and higher levels of ghrelin (a hormone that increases appetite). Lack of sleep may also increase the risk of serious cardiovascular events, including stroke or coronary heart disease. Additionally, sleep affects insulin resistance, and sleep deprivation may increase the risk of developing type 2 diabetes.

Sleep also impacts immune function and inflammation. Lack of sleep may increase the risk of developing irritable bowel disease, gastrointestinal reflux disease, liver disorders, and a wide variety of gastrointestinal diseases. This has been linked to an increase in the amount of inflammatory cytokines. The increase in cytokines causes poor sleep, and poor sleep upregulates the cytokine action. This perpetuates the cycle of sleep dysfunction.

Suffice it to say that water and sleep are a critical part of health, and adequate hydration can help you to overcome some of the initial fatigue, headaches, and brain squirrels that can happen when you cleanse. Drink up every day, and remember to keep track of every glass you drink!

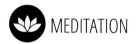 MEDITATION

Hooray! You made it to the end of week one. Congrats! You really are unbeatable. Before we start today's exercise, look back at your notes from Day 1's exercise. What was the number one goal that you determined to be your highest priority? Write it down again and memorize it if you can. You will also need a bit of frankincense essential oil. Portions of the language in this section were adapted from the Aroma Freedom Technique.[11]

TODAY'S MEDITATION

1. Come to a comfortable seated position, and gently invite your eyes to close.
2. Take 3 deep breaths, letting out a small sigh with each exhalation.
3. Envision yourself at the end of this 21-day cleanse with your goal either accomplished or well in progress.
4. How do you feel? Are you proud of your accomplishment? If it is not fully accomplished that is okay! Making lifestyle changes is a commitment for the long term. But maybe even now you can notice a shift in your body. Are you more in tune with your body?
5. Repeat your goal in your head as if it were already a reality. "I am living my healthiest life." "I am filled with healthy cells." "I have a balanced relationship with food." "I am at my healthiest weight." "I am able to control my diabetes." Whatever your goal is, allow it to fill your body as if it were already a reality.
6. If a negative voice arises in your head and says something mean to you that's okay. Sense as deeply as you can where it lives in your body.
7. Once you can identify that place where the negative emotion lives, take a deep inhale of frankincense essential oil from your hand.
8. Breathe deeply into the negative emotion while smelling the frankincense essential oil. If more negativity comes up, that's okay. Just ride the wave of emotion until it passes, and remember that no wave lasts forever.
9. Continue to breathe in the essential oil for as long as you need until you feel that something has shifted.
10. Lower your hands and allow the words of your affirmation to flow to the area of your body where the negative voice lives. Take three deep breaths while repeating your positive affirmation to yourself.

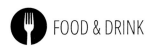 FOOD & DRINK

TODAY'S MENU

B: _____

L: _____

D: _____

REFLECTION ON THE DAY

HOW WAS YOUR SLEEP LAST NIGHT?

The worst, I barely slept   Like a rock

| 1 | 2 | 3 | 4 | 5 | 6 | 7 | 8 | 9 | 10 |

HOW IS YOUR ENERGY TODAY?

I am literally walking dead over here   I could probably run a marathon

| 1 | 2 | 3 | 4 | 5 | 6 | 7 | 8 | 9 | 10 |

THE QUALITY OF YOUR POOP THIS MORNING?

Smelly, severe constipation or diarrhea   Smooth, 10-12 inch masterpiece

| 1 | 2 | 3 | 4 | 5 | 6 | 7 | 8 | 9 | 10 |

HOW ARE YOUR FOOD CRAVINGS TODAY?

Somebody give me a doughnut now   What's to crave? This food is amazing!

| 1 | 2 | 3 | 4 | 5 | 6 | 7 | 8 | 9 | 10 |

REFLECTION ON TODAY

_____

_____

☐ CRUSHED IT!

A KITCHEN WITHOUT A
KNIFE IS NOT A

kitchen

- MASAHARU MORIMOTO -

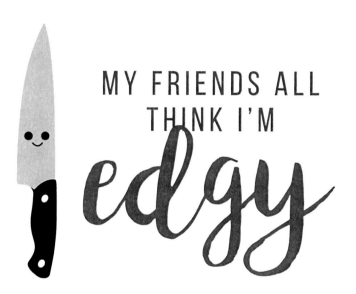

MY FRIENDS ALL THINK I'M *edgy*

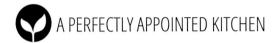 A PERFECTLY APPOINTED KITCHEN

The cleanse requires cooking. Get ready for it, embrace it, and have so much fun cooking. Vegan cooking requires a different set of skills than conventional cooking, and there are certain tools that will make life so much easier around the kitchen.

GOOD 8 OR 10-INCH KNIFE

Nothing in your kitchen will change the ease of cooking more than a high-quality knife. My go-to knife is an 8-inch Wüstof santoku knife, and I use it with almost everything. I occasionally also need a paring knife for small tasks and a 10-inch chef's knife when I really need to leverage weight.

To care for your knives, sharpen them each and every time you use them. Seriously, if your knives are dulled from years of use without sharpening, either send them to be professionally sharpened or invest in new knives. You will not regret it, and your food prep time will significantly decrease (along with the frustration level associated with using dull knives).

Once you are finished using your knife, immediately wash, dry and store it. Nothing breaks my heart more than seeing knives banging around in kitchen utensil drawers. To protect the blades, store them either on a magnet on the wall or in a block. My personal favorite block is from Kapoosh, because it allows you to store many varieties of knives in one block versus having one that is custom designed for specific knives.

SOLID HARDWOOD CUTTING BOARD

Once you have a good knife, why not just grab a nice cutting board to go with it? I know there is concern about bacteria on the board, but thankfully, you are removing meat from the kitchen and this is a major source of bacteria on cutting boards.

To care for your board, always hand wash it immediately after use with warm soapy water. Oil it with a small amount of an edible fatty oil such as almond, olive or fractionated coconut oil. You can add an essential oil like lemon or lemongrass to freshen it while you restore the wood to its natural beauty.

GOOD POTS AND PANS

Whether you choose cast iron, titanium, non-stick, copper, stainless steel or enamel, I don't care. I do care that you LOVE your pots and pans. If you don't love them, get new ones of your choosing.

FOOD PROCESSOR

When cooking vegan, it is next to impossible to survive without a food processor. From blending up burgers and sauces, to shredding blocks of vegan cheese, to slicing massive amounts of vegetables, a food processor makes such a huge difference in food prep time.

Look for one that is dishwasher safe and sized for your needs. If you have a large family, get a larger food processor. I use one from Cuisinart, but there are so many good options to choose from.

IMMERSION BLENDER

If you have a high-powered blender, you will be fine on the cleanse. But an immersion blender blends up soups with less mess than a stand blender. They are so easy to store, dishwasher safe, and powerful enough to blend thick soups. You can even get heavy duty ones if you ever find yourself cooking for a crowd.

A FEW OTHER SMALL THINGS

Be sure you have several nice spatulas, slotted turners, wooden spoons, measuring spoons, stainless steel measuring cups for dry ingredients, and glass measuring cups for wet ingredients.

A FEW MORE OPTIONAL GADGETS

Hand Mixer: I choose a hand mixer instead of a potato masher for potatoes.

Spiralizer: Only need it if you cook the recipes that call for it.

Juicer: You don't have to have it, but man, do I love having one in my kitchen.

Grill Pan: For us city slickers without access to an outdoor barbeque, you can get super creative with a grill pan indoors.

KITCHEN TOOLS SHOPPING LIST

I love today's exercise because a small investment in your kitchen tools can make a huge impact in your success in the cleanse. Make a top 10 list of items that can simplify your cooking routine or a gadget that you would like to try. If you have a very well-appointed kitchen already, consider some fun tea towels or serving spoons. Happy shopping!

1. _____

2. _____

3. _____

4. _____

5. _____

6. _____

7. _____

8. _____

9. _____

10. _____

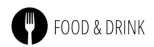 # FOOD & DRINK

TODAY'S MENU

B: _____

L: _____

D: _____

REFLECTION ON THE DAY

HOW WAS YOUR SLEEP LAST NIGHT?

The worst, I barely slept   Like a rock

| 1 | 2 | 3 | 4 | 5 | 6 | 7 | 8 | 9 | 10 |

HOW IS YOUR ENERGY TODAY?

I am literally walking dead over here   I could probably run a marathon

| 1 | 2 | 3 | 4 | 5 | 6 | 7 | 8 | 9 | 10 |

THE QUALITY OF YOUR POOP THIS MORNING?

Smelly, severe constipation or diarrhea   Smooth, 10-12 inch masterpiece

| 1 | 2 | 3 | 4 | 5 | 6 | 7 | 8 | 9 | 10 |

HOW ARE YOUR FOOD CRAVINGS TODAY?

Somebody give me a doughnut now   What's to crave? This food is amazing!

| 1 | 2 | 3 | 4 | 5 | 6 | 7 | 8 | 9 | 10 |

REFLECTION ON TODAY

_____

_____

☐ CRUSHED IT!

HEART DISEASE IS A
FOOD-BORNE

illness

- C A L D W E L L   E S S E L S T Y N -

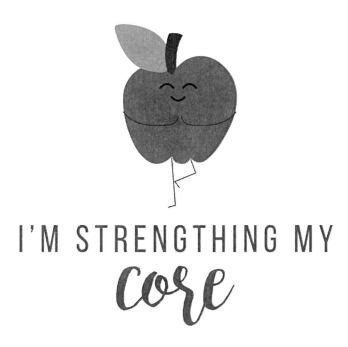

I'M STRENGTHING MY
core

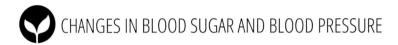

CHANGES IN BLOOD SUGAR AND BLOOD PRESSURE

DIABETES

Blood sugar monitoring is key for people with diabetes. By day 9 of the cleanse, many people with diabetes will notice changes in blood sugar levels. When the brain and body are used to elevated blood sugars, as blood sugars normalize back to non-diabetes levels, many people feel sluggish, tired, or irritable. However, as long as blood sugars are staying within the American Diabetes Association goal for fasting blood sugar (between 80-130 mg/dL) and post-prandial blood sugar (aka 2 hours after a meal) (180 mg/dL),[1] then this is actually a very good sign. The diabetes may be improving with the new way of eating, and the sluggishness and tiredness will pass and improve with time.

It is important to know the signs and symptoms of both high and low blood sugar. Signs of high blood sugar include drinking water without a quench of thirst, excessive urination, headache, difficulty concentrating, blurred vision, fatigue or feeling weak or tired, weight loss or a measured blood sugar of more than 180 mg/dL. Low blood sugar may present with some similar symptoms, such as fatigue, but you may also experience pale skin, shakiness, anxiety, sweating, hunger, or irritability. At extreme levels, people with low blood sugar may experience confusion, abnormal behaviors, visual disturbances, or loss of consciousness. If you experience any of these symptoms, it is important to call your physician and discuss options for increasing or decreasing diabetes medicines.

Let's now talk more generally about how you can protect yourself day to day on the cleanse. The biggest risk is that your blood sugar falls too low. If your blood sugar falls below 70 mg/dL, this indicates low blood sugar. Be sure that you have a fast-acting carb on hand and consume approximately 15 g of juice, sugar, or soda to correct the blood sugar. I acknowledge that this is not the ideal way to eat and certainly not how we eat on the cleanse, but this is different. When people with diabetes have blood sugars that drop low, it is very important to correct them quickly as we do not want them to fall any lower. After you correct this blood sugar, I strongly encourage you to call your physician and discuss lowering doses of diabetes medications, especially sulfonylurea medicines and rapid acting insulin.

If blood sugar falls below 54 mg/dL, it is imperative to treat with 15 g of rapid acting carbohydrates. Check your blood sugar again in 15 minutes. If it is still below 70 mg/dL, call your physician immediately, and discuss a treatment plan. If you cannot get through to your physician, and blood sugar continues to stay low, you may need to go to the hospital or call emergency services.

While there is no specific cutoff for severe hypoglycemia, if you experience any low blood sugar along with severe cognitive impairment, call emergency services immediately.

After any hypoglycemic episode, it is important to discuss the dose of your diabetes medicines with your doctor. If you are noticing these changes now, you may be able to reduce or even eliminate medicines if you are consistent with this diet long term.

BLOOD PRESSURE

Blood pressure may also fall as a result of changing your diet. Normal blood pressure is less than 120/80 mmHg, and blood pressure medicines may be started at 130-139/80-89 mmHg. Low blood pressure is generally considered anything less than 90/60 mmHg.

If you are taking any blood pressure medicines, it is important to recognize the signs of both high and low blood pressure. If you have low blood pressure, you may experience dizziness, lightheadedness (especially upon standing), blurred vision, nausea, fatigue, and inability to concentrate. High blood pressure may have no symptoms at all or may cause dizziness, facial flushing or, in extreme situations, may cause blood spots in the eyes.

I encourage any person with high blood pressure or anyone on blood pressure medicines to have an automatic blood pressure cuff at home. It is a simple device that you can get at your local pharmacy. Ask your pharmacist to help you find your correct size, so you don't get artificially high or low readings. If you ever experience any symptoms of high or low blood sugar, check your blood pressure in the correct way. Sit in a comfortable position for at least five minutes with your legs uncrossed, and your feet flat on the floor. Bring your left arm to chest height and slip on the cuff, and allow the cuff to inflate and automatically give you a reading.

If your blood pressure is below 120/80 mmHg, you may consider asking your physician about adjusting your medicines. However, many physicians choose not to reduce medications until the blood pressure is less than this. Keep up the good work on the cleanse, and you may be able to come off medicines with time and in collaboration with your physician.

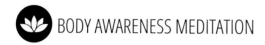 BODY AWARENESS MEDITATION

1. Come to a comfortable seated position, either on the floor or in a chair with your feet firmly placed on the floor. Invite your eyes to close.
2. Slowly take 3 cleansing breaths. In through the nose and out through the mouth, perhaps letting out a little sigh as you exhale. Allow your body to sense the permission to relax.
3. Now allow your breath to return to normal, perhaps a little slower than usual.
4. During this meditation, you are going to scan through your body.
5. As you sit, bring your awareness to the very top of your head. Allow the awareness to drift to your forehead, your brow line, the space between your closed eyelids.
6. Do your nostrils flare as you breathe? Is your tongue on the roof of your mouth, or in the base of your mouth? Are your teeth touching or is there space? Do not aim to judge it or change it, just observe it.
7. Does the air flow freely through your throat? Does your chest rise and fall and expand left and right? Does the air raise the back of your rib cage?
8. Take a deep breath and allow your belly to distend and widen on the inhale and bring the navel back toward the spine on the exhale. Take another deep breath and inhale and exhale, allowing the belly to expand and contract.
9. Next notice your tailbone. Is it squarely placed on the ground or is your pelvis tipped forward or back? Are your hips relaxed? Can you settle your energy any deeper into the earth?
10. Notice your legs. Breathe into your thighs, your kneecaps, your calves. Feel the fluidity of your ankles, feel the space between your toes.
11. Now that we have scanned from head to toe, scan back up from your toes, ankles, calves, knees, thighs, hip sockets, pelvis. Take another breath and allow your belly to distend and contract.
12. Bring your awareness to your rib cage. Feel the vibrations as it expands and contracts.
13. Bring the awareness to the throat, The cheeks, the teeth, the nostrils. Feel the air moving in and out of your nostrils.
14. Are your brows relaxed, are your ears relaxed? Don't feel the need to change it, just be aware.
15. Are the hair sockets on your head relaxed?
16. Scan back down. Notice any areas of tension, any strain, any pain. Simply breath into them and acknowledge that they are a part of you. Breathe in and show love to any bit of the pain. Breathe in and breathe love in the area of pain.
17. Continue this process for three more silent breaths.

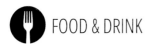 **FOOD & DRINK**

TODAY'S MENU

B: _____

L: _____

D: _____

REFLECTION ON THE DAY

HOW WAS YOUR SLEEP LAST NIGHT?

The worst, I barely slept   Like a rock

| 1 | 2 | 3 | 4 | 5 | 6 | 7 | 8 | 9 | 10 |

HOW IS YOUR ENERGY TODAY?

I am literally walking dead over here   I could probably run a marathon

| 1 | 2 | 3 | 4 | 5 | 6 | 7 | 8 | 9 | 10 |

THE QUALITY OF YOUR POOP THIS MORNING?

Smelly, severe constipation or diarrhea   Smooth, 10-12 inch masterpiece

| 1 | 2 | 3 | 4 | 5 | 6 | 7 | 8 | 9 | 10 |

HOW ARE YOUR FOOD CRAVINGS TODAY?

Somebody give me a doughnut now   What's to crave? This food is amazing!

| 1 | 2 | 3 | 4 | 5 | 6 | 7 | 8 | 9 | 10 |

REFLECTION ON TODAY

_____

_____

☐ CRUSHED IT!

WE SHOULD ALL BE
EATING FRUITS AND
VEGETABLES AS IF OUR
LIVES DEPEND ON IT,
because they do

- MICHAEL GREGER -

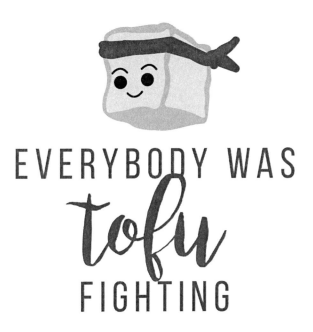

EVERYBODY WAS *tofu* FIGHTING

COMMON QUESTIONS ABOUT PLANT-BASED DIETS

When it comes to research about diets, there is only one true conclusion: it is a gray area without a true black and white. This book admittedly presents data from one angle: that plants are the best way to eat. That said, you can find many opinions to the contrary. You can find plenty of evidence that keto, paleo, carnivorous, and omnivorous diets are healthy. When eating plant-based, there are several questions that come up again and again. Let's review them here.

DO I NEED DAIRY TO GET CALCIUM?

Calcium is great, we all need it, and yes vegans must be conscious to get enough calcium in their diet.

But calcium is not always great. It can quickly become out of balance and lead to worsening of atherosclerotic plaques unless balanced by magnesium. Plant-based sources of calcium such as kale, spinach, chard, and collards also have magnesium, vitamin K, and folate, which can help to balance the potentially deleterious effects of calcium.

This cleanse may also help improve the likelihood that calcium is absorbed and processed correctly. Because we are eliminating caffeine from the diet, we are also increasing the potential for calcium to be absorbed. Caffeine reduces absorption of calcium from foods and beverages and increases excretion.[1,2] Alcohol also decreases the absorption of calcium and inhibits enzymes that convert vitamin D into its storage form.[3,4] While fruits and vegetables high in phytic acid and oxalates may bind calcium and inhibit absorption, diets high in fruits and vegetables also shift the body toward an alkaline state and this reduces calcium excretion.

IS SOY A DANGEROUS FOOD?

This one really depends on who you ask. Soy is one of the most controversial foods out there, especially in recent years. A systematic review assessed five health benefits: relief of menopausal symptoms and prevention of heart disease, breast cancer, prostate cancer, and osteoporosis; and five health risks: increased risk of breast cancer, male hormonal changes and infertility, hypothyroidism, antinutrient content and harmful by-products from processing. In the study, it was revealed that soy-based foods and the isoflavones contained within are likely effective in reducing menopausal symptoms, protecting against breast cancer and heart disease, but not osteoporosis. Data on changes to male fertility are conflicting with some studies showing no effect and others showing potentially deleterious effects. Thyroid function is equally as confusing with some studies showing an increase in thyroid function and others showing a decrease in thyroid function. There is concern that soy-based foods contain high levels of antinutrients that inhibit the absorption of vitamins and minerals. Soaking, cooking, and fermenting may reduce the concentration of these compounds in soy.[5]

I, like the authors of this review, think it is critical to note that there may be a difference between traditionally prepared soy versus the highly processed modern soy. I also wonder if there is allergenicity in play. Soy is one of the big eight allergens. I question if the risk of adverse effects is due to allergic reactions instead of soy itself being a harmful food. I choose to eat soy, as you will see in the recipe section, but I fully support you if you choose not to. You can easily adapt recipes to remove soy-based ingredients. Substitute cauliflower, broccoli, or potatoes for firm tofu. Substitute cashew cream or vegan mayonnaise in recipes that call for silken tofu (just be careful, as you are adding in a larger dose of fat).

DO I NEED MEAT TO GET PROTEIN?

Protein deficiency is extremely rare in isolation. It is almost impossible to be protein deficient without also having a calorie deficiency as well. In the United States, protein deficiency is very rare except as a consequence of pathological conditions or poor medical management of the acutely ill.[6]

It is recommended for the average human adult to ingest 0.8 g protein/kg of body weight per day. So in an average-weight adult (70 kg or 154 lbs.), the recommended protein intake is 56 g/day. But average protein consumption in Americans is higher than that: approximately 90 to 110 g in male and 65 to 70 g in female adolescents and adults (RDA). Newer data suggests that consumption of meat protein is dramatically higher than recommended in men aged 14-70 years of age, and that vegetable protein is significantly under-consumed.[7]

Many people think that you have to eat meat in order to consume enough protein, but this is unlikely to be true. According to a 2014 study comparing dietary intake among vegans, vegetarians, semi-vegetarians (flexitarians), pesco-vegetarians, and omnivores found that each group consumes 82 g, 93 g, 103 g, 100 g, and 112 g, respectively. So even though there was a difference in the amount of protein consumed between the groups, all of the groups well exceeded the recommended daily allowance. This study also demonstrated that omnivores, pesco-vegetarians, partial vegetarians, and vegetarians consumed significantly more cholesterol, saturated fat, and sodium in the diet, and significantly less fiber.[8]

There are alternative protein sources other than meat and dairy that do not require a concomitant dose of excess fat and cholesterol and bring with them a larger dose of cleansing fiber. To ensure that you get enough protein in your vegan diet, include soy-based options (tofu, edamame, or tempeh), lentils and beans (especially black and lima beans), wild rice, chickpeas, chia seeds, steel cut oats, nuts, seeds, and nut butters.

DO HUMANS NEED IRON FROM ANIMAL SOURCES?

Though most people think that it is impossible to get enough iron from a plant-based diet, the same 2014 assessment of more than 1475 vegans, vegetarians, partial vegetarians, pesco-vegetarians, and omnivores mentioned above in the protein data concluded that vegans ate significantly more iron overall and per 1,000 calories in the diet. Interestingly, omnivores ate the least iron both based on absolute intake and per 1,000 calories.[8]

Some contend that even if omnivores eat less iron that it is better absorbed. There are two different forms of iron in foods: heme-iron from meat and non-heme iron from plant-based foods as well as eggs, dairy, and meats. It is known that the absorption of non-heme iron is lower than heme-iron. However, the lower bioavailability also decreases the risk of iron toxicity. Some also posit that non-heme iron has differential absorption depending on the level of iron already in the body.

If you are concerned about not getting enough iron in your diet, be sure to include plenty of high iron vegan foods: spinach, lentils, and pumpkin seeds. Vitamin C increases the absorption of iron, so try a spinach salad with tangerines on top or curried lentils with oranges.

VITAMIN B12

Vegans do have to be careful to get enough vitamin B12 in their diets because this nutrient is primarily found within animal-based foods. The good news is that there are tons of fortified foods and dietary supplements that ensure you do not become nutrient deficient on a vegan diet.

We know that vegans and vegetarians tend to have lower serum vitamin B12 levels than omnivores.[9-11] Recent studies suggest that more than 50% of vegans may be deficient in vitamin B12, and this further indicates the need to supplement on a regular basis.[12]

When selecting a vitamin B12 supplement, I only encourage the use of methylcobalamin instead of cyanocobalamin. Vitamin B12 is a large, watery molecule that has to be bound in the center like a magnet. At the center of a methylcobalamin is a benign methyl group, whereas in the center of a cyanocobalamin, there is a cyanide molecule. Most of the Vitamin B12 at the grocery store is cyanocobalmin, but methylcobalamin can also very easily be found.

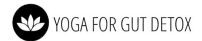 YOGA FOR GUT DETOX

CAT-COW

1. Come to all fours. Stack your knees directly under your hips and your hands directly under your shoulders. As you inhale raise the head and the chest and allow the belly to naturally fall. As you exhale, pull the belly button toward the spine and arc the spine in a natural C-curve with the back of the C toward the ceiling. Repeat, slowly, 8-10 times.

DOWNWARD DOG

2. Following cat-cow, keep your hands and feet in the same spot. As you exhale, reach your hips to the sky. Press your heels into the ground as best you can, but do not move your hands to get your feet on the floor. Gently walk your dog by bending one knee and then another. Stretch your sit bones higher to the ceiling as you walk for five breaths.

TRANSITION

3. After you have walked your dog, stretch both heels back down to the earth again. Look up between your hands and step or jump your feet between your hands. Extend your bum into the air as you inhale, and as you exhale allow all of your upper body's energy to fall to the earth. Inhale and straighten your back ever so slightly, hands reaching toward the earth. Exhale again and allow all energy to melt away from you. Bend your knees, tuck your tail bone forward, and roll up as slowly as you can, as if you are moving through molasses. Allow your head to be the very last thing to come up. Raise your hands over your head as you inhale, and then gently exhale as you bring your hands to a prayer position over your heart. Breathe in and out for three breaths.

SIMPLE TWIST

4. Come to a comfortable cross-legged seated position. Place your left hand behind your back and grab your left knee with your right hand. Take a big inhale, and as you exhale, turn from your torso, with your belly button leading, turning your head last over your left shoulder. As you inhale in the twist, elongate the spine, and with the exhale, twist your body a bit deeper. Take at least 3 deep breaths in this position.

5. Inhale as you turn back to center and gently exhale. Place both hands behind your back, and as you inhale, gently lift the chest and allow the head to drop any amount that is comfortable to you.

6. Now repeat on the other side. Place your right hand behind your back and grab your right knee with your left hand. Take a big inhale, and as you exhale, turn from your torso, with your belly button leading, turning your head last over your right shoulder. As you inhale in the twist, elongate the spine, and with the exhale, twist your body a bit deeper. Take at least 3 deep breaths in this position. Inhale as you turn back to center, and gently exhale. Place both hands behind your back, and as you inhale, gently lift the chest and allow the head to drop any amount that is comfortable to you.

7. As you inhale, bring your head back to a neutral position and bring hands to a comfortable position in your lap.

TRANSITION

8. From the seated cross-legged position, swing your legs in front of you until both feet meet the earth. Tuck the tail bone under and slowly roll, vertebra by vertebra, until your shoulders meet the earth. Allow your head to be the last thing to meet the earth.

SUPINE TWIST

9. Bring both knees into the chest and allow them to gently fall to the right side of your body. Extend both arms into a tee on either side of your body. As is comfortable for you, turn your torso to the left. If comfortable, allow the chest and head to follow to the left, and the knees remain to the right.

10. Take 5 deep breaths.

11. On an inhale, bring your knees back to your chest and roll a bit to give yourself a bit of a back massage.

12. Take another inhale. On an exhale, allow both knees to fall to the left side of your body. Again, extend the arms to a tee. As is comfortable to you, allow your torso to twist to the right, followed by the chest and the head.

13. Take 5 deep breaths.

14. On an inhale, bring your knees back to your chest and roll a bit to give yourself a bit of a back massage.

SAVASANA

15. Allow the legs to extend fully in front of you, and the arms to come to rest, palms up by your sides. Lie still and quiet for at least 1 minute or more. You can quiet the mind entirely or state an affirmation again and again in your mind.

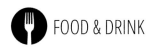 FOOD & DRINK

TODAY'S MENU

B: _____

L: _____

D: _____

REFLECTION ON THE DAY

HOW WAS YOUR SLEEP LAST NIGHT?

The worst, I barely slept   Like a rock

1   2   3   4   5   6   7   8   9   10

HOW IS YOUR ENERGY TODAY?

I am literally walking dead over here   I could probably run a marathon

1   2   3   4   5   6   7   8   9   10

THE QUALITY OF YOUR POOP THIS MORNING?

Smelly, severe constipation or diarrhea   Smooth, 10-12 inch masterpiece

1   2   3   4   5   6   7   8   9   10

HOW ARE YOUR FOOD CRAVINGS TODAY?

Somebody give me a doughnut now   What's to crave? This food is amazing!

1   2   3   4   5   6   7   8   9   10

REFLECTION ON TODAY

_____

_____

☐ CRUSHED IT!

WE MAKE THE WORLD
WE LIVE IN AND SHAPE
OUR OWN
environment

- ORISON SWETT MARDEN -

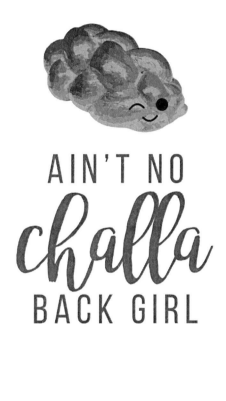

AIN'T NO
challa
BACK GIRL

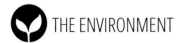 THE ENVIRONMENT

This cleanse is not only good for your body, it is also better for the environment. People who have a vegan diet use significantly less water and less land and generate less carbon dioxide than their omnivorous counterparts. Many people work hard to turn off lights, ride a bike to work, or turn off tap water to save energy and water, but it is less common to consider the impact of what we eat.

The water consumption alone is astonishing: one ⅓ pound hamburger patty requires 660 gallons of water whereas one apple requires 18 gallons of water, and 1 orange 13 gallons. One pound of chicken requires 468 gallons of water versus 216 gallons for a pound of soybeans. One pound of pork requires 576 gallons of water versus 119 gallons for a pound of potatoes. One pound of chocolate requires 3,170 gallons of water versus 1 pound of rice requires 449 gallons. One gallon of coffee requires 880 gallons of water. In fact, if every person in the world drank one cup of coffee per day, it would require 32 trillion gallons of water to supply that caffeine fix.[1]

Consumption of meat and animal products also increases exposure to environmental toxins, and these environmental toxins are known to bioaccumulate. For example, a persistent environmental pollutant such as dioxin may have a low concentration in grass secondary to water runoff. But when the cow eats the grass, it concentrates the toxin in its fat tissues in meat as well as in breastmilk. If a human then eats the meat or drinks the cow's milk, the toxin is then further concentrated in human tissues, and when applicable, in human breastmilk. If a baby is breastfed, the baby will be taking in a very heavily toxin-laden meal.

Dioxins are known endocrine disruptors, and they are a pervasive environmental toxin. The EPA estimates that up to 30% of an adult's overall dioxin exposure is due to consumption of dairy products, and the number increases to 50% in children. The ingestion of high-fat dairy brings with it a cocktail of dioxins, polychlorinated biphenyls and polyfluorinated chemicals, which may result in lower quality semen in men.[2]

Of particular concern for the concentration of environmental toxins is seafood.[3] Seafood has been shown to frequently be contaminated with heavy metals, pollutants, pathogens, and marine toxins.[4-7] One of these risks, pathogens, may be mitigated with proper cooking, handling, and storage of product, but the rest cannot. The most concerning heavy metal in fish is mercury. Mercury is released in the environment by plants and as a byproduct of human activity. It is converted to methylmercury by aquatic organisms. Methylmercury accumulates up the food chain. This means that as you eat increasingly larger and carnivorous fish, the higher the likelihood that the fish is contaminated with mercury.[8] The first documented mercury poisoning due to fish consumption was in the 1950's in Japan, and mercury toxicity has also been associated with consumption of wheat seeds coated in mercury-based fungicides. While adults may have only been mildly or moderately impacted, women who were pregnant at the time of poisoning gave birth to children with severe neurological defects including speech, language and attention problems.[9,10] This has led to stronger warnings against consumption of many fishes during pregnancy and young childhood, especially shark, swordfish, king fish and tile fish.[11]

Mercury is not the only concerning ingredient on the seafood menu. Known carcinogens such as dioxins are present in seafood, and these also are known to bioaccumulate. Even if they do not lead to cancer, polychlorinated biphenyls and dioxins may also cause hormonal changes and changes in fetal development.

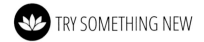 TRY SOMETHING NEW

Today we get to do something fun! We get to think about food. For today's exercise I want you to think of 10 new dishes, fruits, or vegetables that you are excited to try. Perhaps you have been scared to try tofu or a juice recipe; be bold and give it a try. Maybe you want to try an exotic fruit like a papaya, jackfruit, or pomelo. Head over to YouTube and figure out how to cut them and prepare them effectively. Goodness knows, the longer you eat a plant-based diet, the more vegetables you learn to love. When I first started on this plant-based path, I hated olives, mushrooms, tofu, and I had never heard of fennel, aquafaba, or sprouted lentils. Be open minded and give a new food a try!

TEN NEW DISHES, FRUITS, OR VEGETABLES I AM EXCITED TO TRY

1. _____

2. _____

3. _____

4. _____

5. _____

6. _____

7. _____

8. _____

9. _____

10. _____

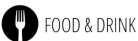

FOOD & DRINK

TODAY'S MENU

B: _____

L: _____

D: _____

REFLECTION ON THE DAY

HOW WAS YOUR SLEEP LAST NIGHT?

The worst, I barely slept   Like a rock

| 1 | 2 | 3 | 4 | 5 | 6 | 7 | 8 | 9 | 10 |

HOW IS YOUR ENERGY TODAY?

I am literally walking dead over here   I could probably run a marathon

| 1 | 2 | 3 | 4 | 5 | 6 | 7 | 8 | 9 | 10 |

THE QUALITY OF YOUR POOP THIS MORNING?

Smelly, severe constipation or diarrhea   Smooth, 10-12 inch masterpiece

| 1 | 2 | 3 | 4 | 5 | 6 | 7 | 8 | 9 | 10 |

HOW ARE YOUR FOOD CRAVINGS TODAY?

Somebody give me a doughnut now   What's to crave? This food is amazing!

| 1 | 2 | 3 | 4 | 5 | 6 | 7 | 8 | 9 | 10 |

REFLECTION ON TODAY

_____

_____

☐ CRUSHED IT!

TRAVEL IS FATAL TO
PREJUDICE, BIGOTRY, AND
narrow-mindedness

- MARK TWAIN -

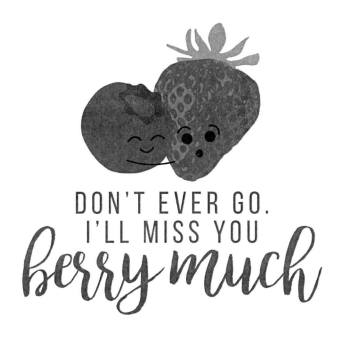

DON'T EVER GO.
I'LL MISS YOU
berry much

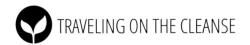# TRAVELING ON THE CLEANSE

I am the first to admit that cleansing on the road is not easy. It takes discipline, heart, and strength. You may face questions from others, and you (honestly) may have to go without a meal until you get to where you have access to food you can eat. I have cried, I have felt defeated, I have had to lean on friends to give me strength. But, I am here to tell you: this is doable. You can do this. You are this strong. You are mighty. Here are some tips to stay strong while traveling:

1. Prep and pack snacks and beverages. Water is a must for travel. I personally am a really unhappy camper unless I have something hot to drink throughout the day, so I always bring peppermint and chamomile teas. For snacks, I love to bring unsalted almonds, dried fruits, rice crackers, seaweed snacks, and granola. I occasionally will succumb to a pre-packaged bar when I am really hungry. Be prepared with snacks and water, lest be at a gas station in the middle of nowhere, and ye regret it.

2. Bring your supplements. I take a lot of supplements, and it is really important that I stay consistent while I am on the road. Bring your multiple vitamin, probiotic, and digestive herbs.

3. Tell the people you are traveling with about the cleanse. Nothing is worse than being on vacation or a work trip when you are on the cleanse than being with someone who is on a completely different wavelength than you. Going with a party patrol to Vegas for the weekend may be really tough, and it will be even tougher if you do not alert your traveling companions. If you are traveling with people who are used to having drinks or cocktails with you, alert them in advance that you will not be drinking on this night out. If you are headed to a family meal, and your dad hasn't missed meat at a meal for 30 years, offer to bring a dish to the get together that suits your needs, and be prepared to answer some questions from people who consider meat a dietary staple.

4. Select restaurants with care. Read menus well, and don't be shy to ask questions. Nothing is nicer than heading to a restaurant that caters to the needs of this cleanse. If you have vegan places in your temporary neighborhood, go check them out. When dining at a conventional restaurant, know that menus have so many ingredients hidden in dishes. Alert your server up front that you would like gluten-free, vegan food with no sugar added, and allow them to make suggestions. If you're at a random pub with friends, you may not have the most amazing choices, but you can also ask for sides of vegetables with no added butter, salad with oil and vinegar, sides of rice, and more. If push comes to shove. . . there are always French fries with malt vinegar. Just saying.

5. Request vegan meals on planes. Man, oh man, what a difference this makes, especially on long flights. I have had perfectly delightful vegan food options on planes. Best of all, it isn't just salads, but warm quinoa dishes, roasted root vegetables, and rice bowls.

6. Deal with stress well. Sometimes, you just have to go with the punches. Don't beat yourself up if you ordered the best you could at a restaurant and there was clearly sugar in the dressing. Don't get flustered if people make fun of you or continue to offer you wine, cheese, or meat. You are stronger than you know.

7. If you know you are headed into the unknown, be sure to eat in advance. While mindful eating is by far my favorite way to eat (see Day 15), when you are traveling it isn't always 100% possible. If I am about to go out for a full day of travel without knowing where my next meal will come from, I will for sure eat before I leave the house or airport, regardless of whether or not I am hungry. This isn't ideal, because ultimately, we want to eat only when we are hungry, but I choose prevention over hangry all day.

8. Never underestimate the power of a good grocery shop. Seriously, head to the grocery store and grab fruit, salad, nuts, or even microwavable soup (I know tons of people hate on the microwave, but after living out of hotel rooms for years; on this cleanse, it can be a game changer to have a bowl of soup ready to go. Again, we give ourselves grace to do our best and forget the rest.)

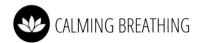 # CALMING BREATHING

Try this simple and calming breathing cycle. It has been shown to decrease cortisol and stress levels. It helps me when I am traveling and face stressful situations.

Gentle breath awareness exercises can energize and reinvigorate the body. Try a cyclic breath.

1. Create a "Y" with your right hand by extending the thumb and pinky finger and tucking the index, middle, and ring fingers down.
2. Cover your left nostril with your pinky finger and take a deep inhalation through the right nostril.
3. Hold your breath and close your thumb over your left nostril, closing both nostrils.
4. Release the pinky finger, and exhale through the left nostril.
5. Inhale through the left nostril.
6. Cover the left nostril with the pinky finger, closing both nostrils.
7. Release the thumb, and exhale through the right nostril.
8. This is one cycle; repeat this cycle at least 3 times.

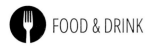 FOOD & DRINK

TODAY'S MENU

B: _____

L: _____

D: _____

REFLECTION ON THE DAY

HOW WAS YOUR SLEEP LAST NIGHT?

The worst, I barely slept   Like a rock

| 1 | 2 | 3 | 4 | 5 | 6 | 7 | 8 | 9 | 10 |

HOW IS YOUR ENERGY TODAY?

I am literally walking dead over here   I could probably run a marathon

| 1 | 2 | 3 | 4 | 5 | 6 | 7 | 8 | 9 | 10 |

THE QUALITY OF YOUR POOP THIS MORNING?

Smelly, severe constipation or diarrhea   Smooth, 10-12 inch masterpiece

| 1 | 2 | 3 | 4 | 5 | 6 | 7 | 8 | 9 | 10 |

HOW ARE YOUR FOOD CRAVINGS TODAY?

Somebody give me a doughnut now   What's to crave? This food is amazing!

| 1 | 2 | 3 | 4 | 5 | 6 | 7 | 8 | 9 | 10 |

REFLECTION ON TODAY

_____

_____

☐ CRUSHED IT!

FOR EVERY DISCIPLINED
EFFORT, THERE IS A

multiple reward

- JIM ROHN -

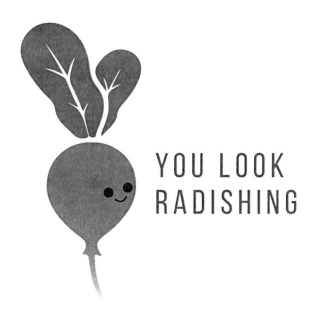

YOU LOOK
RADISHING

CELEBRATING IN THE MIDDLE OF A CLEANSE

We've been at this for almost two weeks, and it is important to celebrate the small victories each day. Often, we reach for a food reward during holidays and other times of celebration, and it has become commonplace to only look to food as a reward. Let's discuss some rewards that we can use instead food.

1. Something for the kitchen. Nothing is better to me than a much needed and desired kitchen instrument. A fancy knife can be life changing in a vegan kitchen. A new juicer can help you get more nutrition and yield out of your fruits and vegetables. A food processor can cut prep time down dramatically. A new set of beautiful napkins or a gorgeous new set of plates can transform your table. And for goodness sake, replace annoying gadgets like rusty can openers, cracked cutting boards, or dull vegetable peelers. What have you been craving in your kitchen that would be both useful and fun to buy?

2. Pampering. Chances are you may be seeing some changes in your body at this point. Perhaps you have gotten over some initial muscle cramps or fatigue during week one. Maybe your skin is clearer. Sounds like a perfect excuse for a massage, facial, or a little bit of waxing to make you feel sexy. Pick your favorite spa service and make an appointment to take care of you.

3. A night out. Ever been to a musical or the theatre? What about to see your favorite sports team? To see the band you've loved for years? Now's the time to grab tickets for yourself and a loved one.

4. Push even further. Ready to go to another level with your health and wellness? Book a series of meditation sessions or yoga classes. Try rock climbing, grab a new workout outfit, or pick up a cookbook that supports your healthy choices.

5. Grab a treatment. Book a visit to the acupuncturist, a session with a chiropractor, or a sign up for a reiki session. Take an intentional break from your day and recharge.

6. Unapologetic me time. Take a day to stay in your favorite place. Whether reading in your favorite chair, getting a manicure, or out on a hike, take time to celebrate in the way that is exactly what you want.

7. Do something you have never done. Or even better, something that you couldn't do when you first started. Go on a family bike ride, play catch with a child, or head to a museum, park, or beach. Is there a weekend getaway you have always wanted to take? Pick something you have always wanted to do and make plans.

8. Indulge in a daily luxury. Hate cleaning? Book a housekeeper. Hate laundry? Send it out for laundering. Tired of shopping for groceries? Get them delivered. Want a break from planning meals? Order a meal prep delivery box. Something simple that takes a small burden off of you can be a huge reward.

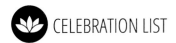 CELEBRATION LIST

Make a top 10 list of the favorite things you would like to do to celebrate your successes so far. From there, pick your favorite and go treat yourself! After you have your top 10 list, you can always come back to this page. When you are struggling to stay strong, set a goal for which you will reward yourself again with one more item on this list.

1. _____

2. _____

3. _____

4. _____

5. _____

6. _____

7. _____

8. _____

9. _____

10. _____

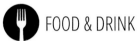 FOOD & DRINK

TODAY'S MENU

B: _____

L: _____

D: _____

⭕ REFLECTION ON THE DAY

HOW WAS YOUR SLEEP LAST NIGHT?

The worst, I barely slept   Like a rock

1   2   3   4   5   6   7   8   9   10

HOW IS YOUR ENERGY TODAY?

I am literally walking dead over here   I could probably run a marathon

1   2   3   4   5   6   7   8   9   10

THE QUALITY OF YOUR POOP THIS MORNING?

Smelly, severe constipation or diarrhea   Smooth, 10-12 inch masterpiece

1   2   3   4   5   6   7   8   9   10

HOW ARE YOUR FOOD CRAVINGS TODAY?

Somebody give me a doughnut now   What's to crave? This food is amazing!

1   2   3   4   5   6   7   8   9   10

REFLECTION ON TODAY

_____

_____

☐ CRUSHED IT!

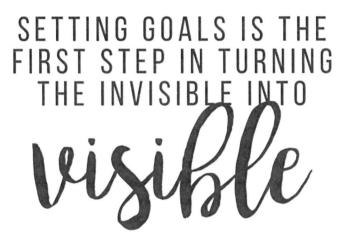

SETTING GOALS IS THE
FIRST STEP IN TURNING
THE INVISIBLE INTO

visible

- T O N Y   R O B B I N S -

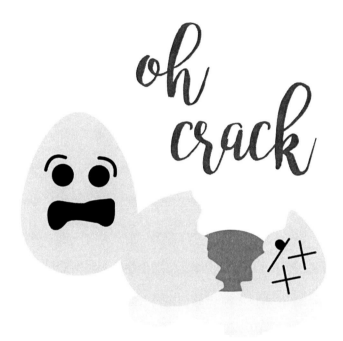

WHY AVOID MEAT AND ANIMAL PRODUCTS, PART 2

It may seem like overkill to have two chapters on the reasons for avoiding meat and animal products, but there is so much data it was impossible for me to get it all in one chapter. So let's talk now about bacteria and hormones in animal products.

BACTERIA IN ANIMAL PRODUCTS

Foodborne illnesses are sometimes transmitted via meat and animal products. There are more than 250 foodborne diseases, caused by bacteria such as *Salmonella, Staphylococcus aureus, Campylobacter, Clostridium, Listeria,* and *Vibrio,* viruses such as norovirus, and infectious protein prions in variant Creutzfeldt-Jakob disease (aka Mad Cow Disease).[1] Older adults, infants, and people with weakened immune systems are at risk for more serious and potentially life-threatening disease.

The Centers for Disease Control (CDC) estimates that 1.2 million people are made ill by *Salmonella,* causing 450 deaths each year. Of particular concern for *Salmonella* are eggs, because 1 in every 20,000 is contaminated. The CDC suggests against the consumption of raw egg products for anyone due to the risk of *Salmonella* infection.

ANIMAL PRODUCTS AND HORMONES

There are many people who worry about the consumption of soy-based products because of the risk of phytoestrogens. Yet many do not stop to question the hormones in animal-based ingredients.

There is no meat out there that does not contain hormones,[2] and these are at least 10,000 times more potent than environmental xenoestrogens.[3] This is particularly important because the hormones in animals are the exact same as our own. There are many meats labeled as hormone-free, but this means that they have had no hormones added. It does not mean that they are without hormones. Since they are animals, any hormone they have in their bodies will be consumed along with the meat. Almost every chicken sold in grocery stores is female, so consumption of chicken (as well as eggs) is especially laden with estrogens,[4] whereas in this same study no estrogens could be found in vegetable foods.

While meat and eggs are major sources of estrogens in the diet, the largest sources are milk and dairy products. Consumption of 300 mL of milk per day can provide up to 10 g of estrogen, and this is 4,000 times the intake of environmental toxins. Exposure to estrogen may have negative health consequences. For example, cheese intake has been specifically shown to decrease sperm concentration, as well as producing abnormal sperm shape and movement.[5,6]

Furthermore, the excretion of hormones into the urine and feces by food animals may contribute up to 90% of total estrogens in the water supply.[7] The addition of hormones to poultry is banned by US law; the estrogen levels in the droppings of poultry is so high that when farmers feed their animals poultry manure to save on cost, it can lead to premature development. The estrogen levels are so high in fact that the estrogen may create a complete carcinogen as it exerts both tumor-initiating and tumor-promoting effects in any animal that consumes it.[8]

While the addition of hormones into poultry is banned, 33% of beef manufacturers in the U.S. add either natural or synthetic estrogens, testosterone, and progesterones to stimulate growth while the animals are still nursing).[9] Addition of hormones to beef cattle has been banned in Europe for 25 years because of evidence that it caused reproductive harm.[10]

So why is it so common to inject hormones into beef cattle, but not chickens? That is because over the course of 50 years, chickens have been subject to an intentional genetic selection pressure that has led to favoring larger birds. From 1957-2007, the average size of a chicken increased 400%.[11] But this breeding program has also lead to several unintentional consequences such as: sexual dimorphism, skeletal defects, metabolic disorders, and altered immune function in animals.[12-15] So we now have evidence in two species that either the addition of hormones or genetic pressure favoring large birds may lead to unintended health consequences in both animals and humans.

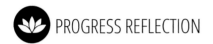 PROGRESS REFLECTION

Write a letter to your present self and reflect on where you have been and where you still hope to go.

You are now starting into week 3 of the cleanse. Let's take a moment to reflect on your progress and the week ahead.

1. List 3 reasons you are grateful you are still on the cleanse.

_____

2. What have been your successes so far?

_____

3. How did you celebrate your success?

_____

4. What would you still like to accomplish in the last week?

_____

5. What are you most looking forward to this week?

_____

6. What challenges do you anticipate this week?

_____

7. What will you do when challenges arise?

_____

8. List 3 new foods you are most excited to try.

_____

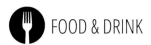 FOOD & DRINK

TODAY'S MENU

B: _____

L: _____

D: _____

REFLECTION ON THE DAY

HOW WAS YOUR SLEEP LAST NIGHT?

The worst, I barely slept   Like a rock

1   2   3   4   5   6   7   8   9   10

HOW IS YOUR ENERGY TODAY?

I am literally walking dead over here   I could probably run a marathon

1   2   3   4   5   6   7   8   9   10

THE QUALITY OF YOUR POOP THIS MORNING?

Smelly, severe constipation or diarrhea   Smooth, 10-12 inch masterpiece

1   2   3   4   5   6   7   8   9   10

HOW ARE YOUR FOOD CRAVINGS TODAY?

Somebody give me a doughnut now   What's to crave? This food is amazing!

1   2   3   4   5   6   7   8   9   10

REFLECTION ON TODAY

_____

_____

☐ CRUSHED IT!

YOU ARE NOT A MISTAKE.
YOU ARE NOT A PROBLEM TO
BE SOLVED. BUT YOU WON'T
DISCOVER THIS UNTIL YOU ARE
WILLING TO STOP BANGING YOUR
HEAD AGAINST THE WALL OF
SHAMING AND CAGING AND
FEARING YOURSELF.

- GENEEN ROTH -

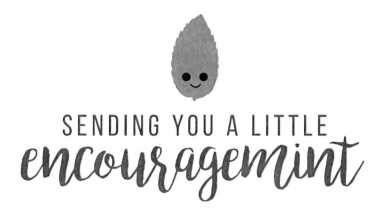

SENDING YOU A LITTLE
encouragemint

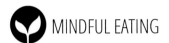 MINDFUL EATING

Geneen Roth changed my life with her writings, especially her work *Women, Food and God*. She contends that it is not so much about what we eat as how we eat it, and that our entire relationship with ourselves, others, and the universe is right there on our plate. The way that you eat is inseparable from your core beliefs about being alive. The way that you eat tells more about you than all of your other actions. Do you eat to nourish your body or as a form of abuse and punishment? She contends that when you can take a difficult look at the ways you use food to soothe, numb or distract yourself, you can uncover deeper spirituality, self-love and a brightness that is already in you, waiting to be discovered.[1]

This book is a testament to mindful eating, because when we are mindful we take back control from food, and our relationship with both food and ourselves improves.

There are so many times that we sit down to a plate of food without any concept of whether or not we are really hungry. We eat out of boredom, celebration, guilt, loneliness, and a million reasons other than true hunger. We use food to abuse ourselves on a daily, ongoing basis. There are times we feel healthiness is a battle between hamburgers and salads. We literally obsess over chocolate cake and pizza at kid's birthday parties, and shame ourselves for 'giving in' when we should be dieting. We mistakenly think the key to having that perfect body is a matter of will-power. But like everything else in the world there is only one answer: awareness and love.

Awareness is the starting point, and to be aware you must fully land in your body. Before you start to eat, ask yourself: "Am I truly hungry?" Or "Am I bored, sad, annoyed, celebrating, craving sugar, craving a friend?" If it is any one of those emotions, I encourage you, find something, anything to do other than eat. Paint a picture, go to a movie, call an old friend, go to a yoga class. If you're not genuinely hungry. . . you don't get to eat. When we eat, we cannot eat out of obsession, we must eat out of awareness. Geneen makes a powerful argument for why diets don't work as a means to achieve weight loss. When you simply try to restrict food intake, and ignore the battle between awareness and obsession, obsession inevitably wins. If the chocolate cake across the room from you seems like it has arms, remember, "I can have that food, I am choosing not to eat it."

At this point in the cleanse, some people discover that they eat mindlessly. Yes, they will adhere to the cleanse dietary restrictions, but if you find yourself reaching for food when you don't even know if you're hungry, these next two days are for you. Today is the first of two days of mindful eating exercises. I encourage you to do both at least once and really take inventory of the awareness and obsession we have with food. Be kind to yourself with every single bite.

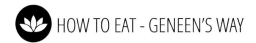 HOW TO EAT - GENEEN'S WAY

For today's exercise, we will use Geneen's Guidance on how to eat:

EAT WHEN YOU ARE HUNGRY.

1. Ask yourself, "How hungry am I, on a scale of 1-10?" With 1 being not hungry at all and 10 being the hungriest I have ever been.
2. If you are hungry, ask yourself "What is the most delicious (cleanse-approved) thing I can think of to eat right now?"
3. Make that food. And:

   - Eat sitting down in a calm environment. This does not include the car.
   - Eat without distractions. Distractions include radio, television, newspapers, books, intense or anxiety-producing conversations or music.
   - Eat what your body wants.
   - Eat until you are satisfied.
   - With every bite, ask yourself, "How hungry am I, on a scale of 1-10?" With 1 being not hungry at all and 10 being the hungriest I have ever been. Stop eating before you are stuffed full.
   - Eat (with the intention of being) in full view of others.
   - Eat with enjoyment, gusto and pleasure.

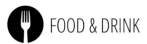 FOOD & DRINK

TODAY'S MENU

B: _____

L: _____

D: _____

REFLECTION ON THE DAY

HOW WAS YOUR SLEEP LAST NIGHT?

The worst, I barely slept   Like a rock

1   2   3   4   5   6   7   8   9   10

HOW IS YOUR ENERGY TODAY?

I am literally walking dead over here   I could probably run a marathon

1   2   3   4   5   6   7   8   9   10

THE QUALITY OF YOUR POOP THIS MORNING?

Smelly, severe constipation or diarrhea   Smooth, 10-12 inch masterpiece

1   2   3   4   5   6   7   8   9   10

HOW ARE YOUR FOOD CRAVINGS TODAY?

Somebody give me a doughnut now   What's to crave? This food is amazing!

1   2   3   4   5   6   7   8   9   10

REFLECTION ON TODAY

_____

_____

☐ CRUSHED IT!

PERSISTENCE GUARANTEES
THAT RESULTS ARE

inevitable

- PARAMAHANSA YOGANANDA -

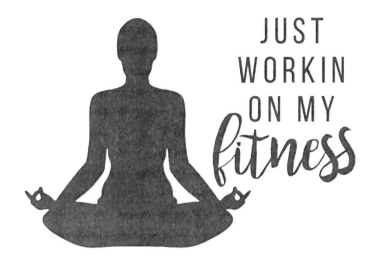

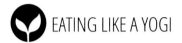 # EATING LIKE A YOGI

Today we go through another exercise about eating with intention and mindfulness. This is an adaptation of an exercise that was taught to me by my colleague Jodie Meschuk, who learned it during her training as a yoga teacher. Eating like a yogi is about using food as a connection with one's soul and the universe around us versus using food solely as a way to satisfy hunger. As with most mindful eating practices, step one of the process is to listen to the body and to first determine if true hunger exists before any food is ingested.

Then we start to explore the universe in front of us on our plate: listen to the food in front of you. Can you sense the origins of the food? What about the soil in which it was grown? The farmer who nurtured the seed? The cultivator who grew the food? The harvester who picked the food? What about the sun and water that went into the growing process? If your food does not possess any of the qualities of nature, perhaps it is not a food that should be on your plate. And I say this with the understanding that on this cleanse, we do consume processed food such as tempeh, tofu, vegetable cheeses, etc. This is a great day to choose to avoid some of these foods and to choose more live foods.

Many yogis are vegan, vegetarian, gluten-free or pescatarian. There is no rule against eating meat when living a yogi lifestyle but be sure you are doing it with exceptionally clear intention and gratitude. Following are some additional questions to consider asking if after the cleanse you choose to resume consuming meat. How was this animal raised? How was it slaughtered? Did the animal have access to clean water, fresh air, and food that is close to what it would eat in the wild? If you don't know the answers to these questions, this may not be an animal you choose to add to your plate.

Many yogis eat according Ayurvedic eating principles as well. In Ayurvedic traditions, there are three body types, or doshas. The Kapha is the largest body type, typically with wide hips and shoulders, thick hair, good physical stamina, and sluggish digestion. People with this energy are reliable, steady and slow to learn but have excellent memories. The diet should be low in fat, sweets, and salt, and high in vegetables, spices, and high fiber foods such as legumes, as these will help to speed digestion. When out of balance, Kapha people can get poor circulation and may be obese.

The Pitta dosha is the medium build. People with this energy tend to have good muscle tone, tend to feel warm all the time, and have excellent digestion. Pitta people are intelligent, focused, and ambitious. They can suffer from inflammatory conditions when out of balance. The diet should avoid hot spices, alcohol, coffee, vinegar and acidic foods. Cooling vegetables like cucumbers, kale and lettuce are excellent additions to the diet.

The final dosha is Vata, and this is the smallest body type. Vata people are thin with prominent bones, find it difficult to gain weight, tend to be cold all the time, and have small muscles. They learn fast and forget things easily, and are creative and excitable. When out of balance, Vata people have a lot of bloating and constipation, insomnia, and fatigue. It is recommended to avoid dry/crunchy foods, carbonated beverages, and cold/raw vegetables. Ideally, Vata people eat warm, cooked foods, especially soup, congee, oatmeal, and cooked vegetables.

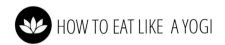 # HOW TO EAT LIKE A YOGI

Today we will eat like a yogi. I encourage you to do at least one full meal in this way. Eat three meals per day with little to no snacking in between, as this is thought to maximize nutrient absorption.

1. Breakfast is comprised primarily of grains such as soaked oats and nuts, and chia seeds. Warm beverages such as teas are suggested, especially turmeric tea.

2. Lunch is comprised of raw vegetables and salads.

3. Dinner is the best time to eat cooked foods, including earthy foods, like sweet potatoes, as well as proteins.

4. Feet are both firmly grounded to the earth, and posture is upright and straight.

5. The yogi meal is typically consumed in silence. The silence may be only a portion of one meal, a full day, or may extend for several weeks. In my experience, eating in silence is much more pleasurable when you smile. It can be quite depressing if you are sitting with slouched body language. Remember your posture. I acknowledge that this may be challenging with children and talkative adults. If you have talkative members of your household, be sure that you have prepared them in advance that you will be eating in this way and give permission for people to get up from the table between bites to quickly grab a napkin, condiment or additional foods when needed. Only leave the table in between bites.

6. Chewing is a critical piece of the meal. Every bit of food should be chewed 15-20 times at a minimum to soothe and ease digestion. Any utensils should be placed on the table between each bite.

7. Some people choose to say an affirmation between each bite to further slow the food consumption process.

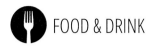 FOOD & DRINK

TODAY'S MENU

B: _____

L: _____

D: _____

REFLECTION ON THE DAY

HOW WAS YOUR SLEEP LAST NIGHT?

The worst, I barely slept   Like a rock

| 1 | 2 | 3 | 4 | 5 | 6 | 7 | 8 | 9 | 10 |

HOW IS YOUR ENERGY TODAY?

I am literally walking dead over here   I could probably run a marathon

| 1 | 2 | 3 | 4 | 5 | 6 | 7 | 8 | 9 | 10 |

THE QUALITY OF YOUR POOP THIS MORNING?

Smelly, severe constipation or diarrhea   Smooth, 10-12 inch masterpiece

| 1 | 2 | 3 | 4 | 5 | 6 | 7 | 8 | 9 | 10 |

HOW ARE YOUR FOOD CRAVINGS TODAY?

Somebody give me a doughnut now   What's to crave? This food is amazing!

| 1 | 2 | 3 | 4 | 5 | 6 | 7 | 8 | 9 | 10 |

REFLECTION ON TODAY

_____

_____

☐ CRUSHED IT!

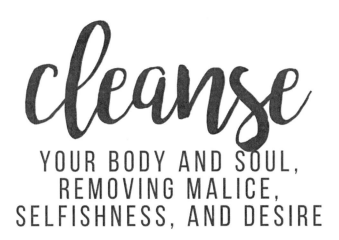

cleanse

YOUR BODY AND SOUL,
REMOVING MALICE,
SELFISHNESS, AND DESIRE

- M O R I H E I   U E S H I B A -

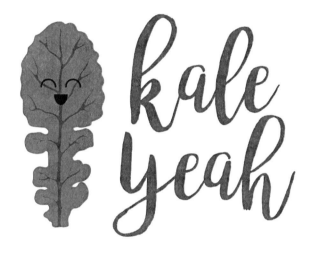

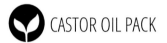 CASTOR OIL PACK

Today begins a 3-day series of optional cleanses. The gentlest is the castor oil pack (today's exercise), while the gallbladder cleanse and coffee enemas are a bit more assertive. Please read through the safety precautions carefully.

One of my favorite ways to relax and recharge is using a castor oil pack. Historical textbooks list castor oil as one of the oldest ways to support health with citations dating back to 1550 BC in Egypt, thousands of years in India and China, and it was deemed the Palma Christa in medieval Europe.

WHAT IS CASTOR OIL?

Castor oil and its major constituent, ricinoleic acid, an unsaturated omega-9 fatty acid, have been researched for pain killing, anti-inflammatory, laxative, and uterine relaxation effects. Let's first look at the anti-inflammatory effects. Castor oil increases the levels of T-11 lymphocytes in the top layers of the skin, and this is thought to give castor oil its anti-inflammatory effects. Castor oil also increases prostaglandin E2 and activates the EP3 prostanoid receptor, and this may be responsible for the induction of labor in pregnant women.

Castor oil packs may also bring additional blood to the liver and reduce pain. The heat from a castor oil pack increases blood flow and may improve oxygenation to target tissues. Castor oil activates the VR1 receptor similarly to the over-the-counter pain reliever capsaicin, and this may account for its analgesic effects.

Castor oil has a strong laxative effect that comes from the ricinoleic acid activating peristalsis (the rhythmic movement of the gut) in the small intestine. While castor oil packs have not been shown to increase the number of bowel movements in elderly people with chronic constipation, they can help to decrease fecal consistency scores, straining during defecation, and perception of complete evacuation during defecation.[1]

Castor oil may also have liver-protecting, antioxidant, mercury scavenging, and antimicrobial effects.

WHAT IS A CASTOR OIL PACK?

Castor oil packs are a gentle way to detoxify the liver or support reproductive health using a topical application of castor oil. You saturate a wool flannel in castor oil, lay it either on top of the liver (under the right breast) or on the uterus, and then use a hot water bottle to provide heat. The heat brings fresh blood to the liver or uterus, and the castor oil itself protects the liver and relaxes the uterus. Today we will complete a castor oil pack.

SAFETY PRECAUTIONS

1. During menstruation, castor oil packs may ease menstrual cramps. However, you may find that menstrual blood flow is increased following a castor oil pack.
2. When trying to become pregnant, the increased blood flow to the uterus may support the ability to become pregnant, but the heat may interfere with sperm viability.
3. Do not use castor oil packs during pregnancy as it is well known to relax the uterus and may cause miscarriage. It is very strongly recommended to avoid castor oil by mouth at any point during pregnancy as it is well documented to have the potential to induce labor.[2]
4. Castor oil packs have been shown to be safe in women with uterine fibroids.
5. Do not use castor oil packs if bleeding internally, if you have an active infection, if you have excessive gas, or if you have a colon malformation.

HOW TO DO A CASTOR OIL PACK

For today's exercise, let's do a castor oil pack! First gather supplies:

- Wool flannel large enough to cover the liver. Alternatively, you may choose to get a larger piece of wool that can cover the entire abdomen.
- Organic, cold pressed castor oil
- Plastic wrap
- Hot water bottle
- Towel that you don't mind getting oily
- Storage container for wool flannel once finished with pack (a mason jar or plastic bag will do just fine)

DIRECTIONS:

1. Warm water on the stove until almost boiling. Lay an old towel that you don't mind getting stained on bed or couch.
2. Stretch plastic wrap over towel and lay out piece of wool flannel.
3. Saturate the flannel in castor oil (you want it fully saturated, but not dripping).
4. Once water is warm, fill hot water bottle.
5. Place wool flannel and plastic wrap on top of liver or uterus. Be sure that as much of the flannel is covered with plastic wrap as possible.
6. Lie down on towel and place warm water bottle on top of liver or uterus.
7. Relax for 20-30 minutes or longer. Repeat this procedure as often as desired.
8. .Once finished, discard water and plastic wrap. Rub excess castor oil into skin and wash hands. Place wool flannel in mason jar or plastic bag and store in the refrigerator. You can reuse the wool flannel dozens of times. Add a bit more castor oil each time.

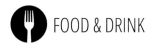 FOOD & DRINK

TODAY'S MENU

B: _____

L: _____

D: _____

REFLECTION ON THE DAY

HOW WAS YOUR SLEEP LAST NIGHT?

The worst, I barely slept   Like a rock

| 1 | 2 | 3 | 4 | 5 | 6 | 7 | 8 | 9 | 10 |

HOW IS YOUR ENERGY TODAY?

I am literally walking dead over here   I could probably run a marathon

| 1 | 2 | 3 | 4 | 5 | 6 | 7 | 8 | 9 | 10 |

THE QUALITY OF YOUR POOP THIS MORNING?

Smelly, severe constipation or diarrhea   Smooth, 10-12 inch masterpiece

| 1 | 2 | 3 | 4 | 5 | 6 | 7 | 8 | 9 | 10 |

HOW ARE YOUR FOOD CRAVINGS TODAY?

Somebody give me a doughnut now   What's to crave? This food is amazing!

| 1 | 2 | 3 | 4 | 5 | 6 | 7 | 8 | 9 | 10 |

REFLECTION ON TODAY

_____

_____

☐ CRUSHED IT!

DON'T WATCH THE CLOCK;
DO WHAT IT DOES.

keep going

- SAM LEVENSON -

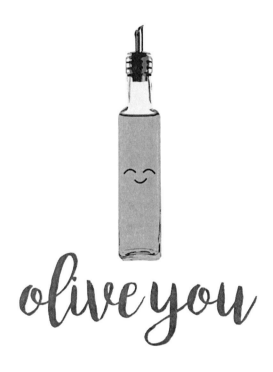

olive you

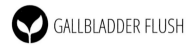 GALLBLADDER FLUSH

This gallbladder flush comes from the book that has done more to inform my opinions on natural products than any other publication: *Healing with Whole Foods* by Paul Pitchford.[1] This is not exactly a mild cleanse, and I do not recommend it for anyone without a gallbladder (as it is unnecessary). It takes discipline to get through the day, but honestly, this is much easier than you might think it will be. You are getting plenty of calories through the day. With water and apples, you are also getting plenty of hydration. I recommend that you have the next morning off from work or other appointments in case you have a lot of bowel movements following this flush.

I will be honest, there is not great scientific data to suggest this gallbladder flush works, but I have heard and observed from a lot of people that it works well for them. Theoretically, problems associated with a low functioning gallbladder include: inflammation of the gallbladder and bile ducts, muscular spasms and/or poor contraction of the gallbladder wall, stones forming in the gallbladder and/or bile ducts, obstruction to the free flow of bile. This can lead to upper abdominal pain, which is primarily treated with surgery. The problem with surgery is that it doesn't always solve the upper abdominal pain, and, I mean… it is surgery.

Why do we need to cleanse the gallbladder? The function of the gallbladder is to store and concentrate bile, which is a digestive enzyme made by the liver. Bile is important for the digestion of fats, and it also collects waste products from the liver and passes them into the small intestine. People with gallstones rarely feel any symptoms until the stones are large enough to obstruct flow of bile through the biliary system. Human survival is possible without a gallbladder, as the bile can reach the small intestine via alternate routes, but there is not as much bile as there was previously. Though most people do not notice a change in digestion following gallbladder removal, bile is critical for the digestion and absorption of fats and fat-soluble vitamins. There may theoretically be a change in absorption even if it is unnoticed.

The middle of this cleanse is the perfect time to flush the gallbladder because we know that, compared to omnivores, vegetarians have a lower risk of gallstones and gallbladder disease.[2]

There are only a couple of ingredients in the gallbladder cleanse: apples, olive oil, lemon juice, and (if you choose) Epsom salts. Apple juice contains malic acid that dissolves the cohesion between gallbladder stones. Olive oil helps the gallbladder squeeze itself to push out gallstones. Lemon juice cuts the flavor of olive oil and makes it more palatable. Epsom salts relax the bile duct to allow stones to pass more easily. Some people will experience large stones that come out, and others choose to use a flashlight to look for bright green, heavy stones in the stool. Some people may feel sick for a day or two afterward, and this may be an indication of an underlying parasitic infection.

SAFETY PRECAUTIONS

1. There are some risks associated with gallbladder flushing. Some people experience nausea, vomiting, diarrhea, or abdominal pain.
2. If you have any type of gastrointestinal disorder or are pregnant or nursing, please consult with your physician before beginning.
3. This is not recommended for people who do not have a gallbladder, as it is unlikely to help.

LET'S DO A GALLBLADDER FLUSH

DIRECTIONS:

1. Beginning in the morning and throughout the day, only consume green apples throughout the day. Eat as many as you like, but at least 4-5.

2. At bedtime, warm ⅔ cup olive oil to body temperature and add ⅓ cup lemon juice. Slowly drink the entire mixture. Some people choose to drink 8 oz. of water blended with 1 tablespoon Epsom salts before the oil. This is optional. It can help to relax the gallbladder sphincter, but really doesn't taste great.

3. Immediately go to bed. Sleep on your right side with your right knee pulled up to your chest.

4. Alternatively, you can do a gentler version of this cleanse. For 5 consecutive days, first thing in the morning on an empty stomach, ingest two tablespoons of olive oil followed by two tablespoons of lemon juice.

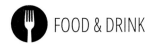 FOOD & DRINK

TODAY'S MENU

B: _____

L: _____

D: _____

REFLECTION ON THE DAY

HOW WAS YOUR SLEEP LAST NIGHT?

The worst, I barely slept   Like a rock

| 1 | 2 | 3 | 4 | 5 | 6 | 7 | 8 | 9 | 10 |

HOW IS YOUR ENERGY TODAY?

I am literally walking dead over here   I could probably run a marathon

| 1 | 2 | 3 | 4 | 5 | 6 | 7 | 8 | 9 | 10 |

THE QUALITY OF YOUR POOP THIS MORNING?

Smelly, severe constipation or diarrhea   Smooth, 10-12 inch masterpiece

| 1 | 2 | 3 | 4 | 5 | 6 | 7 | 8 | 9 | 10 |

HOW ARE YOUR FOOD CRAVINGS TODAY?

Somebody give me a doughnut now   What's to crave? This food is amazing!

| 1 | 2 | 3 | 4 | 5 | 6 | 7 | 8 | 9 | 10 |

REFLECTION ON TODAY

_____

_____

☐ CRUSHED IT!

strive for
progress
NOT PERFETION

- U N K N O W N -

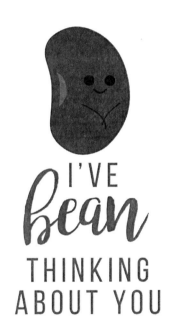

I'VE *bean* THINKING ABOUT YOU

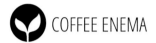 COFFEE ENEMA

The notion of colon cleansing is nothing new; accounts actually date back to Ancient Egypt. Coffee enemas were conceptualized in 1917 and were heavily researched in the 1920's. Coffee enemas are a long-standing part of the Gerson Method used to treat cancers.[1] According to Gerson, coffee enemas have been shown to aid in detoxification of the liver, expel bile juice, reduce abdominal pain, and release toxic matter. This is because they can dilate the bile ducts and allow the liver to release byproducts through the intestinal tract.[2] They may be an effective portion in the treatment of acute and chronic inflammatory disease. Coffee enemas may also have a role in treating cancer pain and removing parasites.

Just like the gallbladder cleanse, there is not a ton of excellent evidence that coffee enemas work. In fact, the data is actually quite poor. But from my own experience, coffee enemas can be transformative and more powerful than warm water enemas.

From what data we do have, we know the following. Proponents of coffee enemas claim they increase the body's ability to detoxify itself. Cafestol diacetate found in coffee is a potent inducer of glutathione S-transferase (GST) in the animal liver and small bowel mucosa. GST helps the body to attach its master detoxifier, glutathione, to toxins, making them water-soluble. They can then be eliminated from the body. It also serves an enzymatic function that helps to release bile from the gallbladder and move it into the intestines. Cafestol is one of two GST-inducers found in coffee. Coffee itself is known to induce GST, and when fed green as a food additive, could enhance GST six-fold in the liver and seven-fold in the small bowel.

The procedure for a coffee enema is simple, but the safety precautions cannot be ignored. People have suffered exceptional harm from coffee enemas that are too warm.[3] Caffeine absorption can be rapid and intoxicating, so be sure to lay on your right side. This is especially important since we have not been consuming caffeine for over two weeks now. Ensure that your enema supplies are clean, as they may harbor infectious bacteria that cause sepsis. Do not overuse coffee enemas, as they can cause electrolyte imbalances and dehydration.[4]

SAFETY PRECAUTIONS

1. Talk to a physician before starting a new health and wellness routine. It is controversial whether enemas should be used during pregnancy. Be sure to discuss with your physician or midwife. Do not use more than daily, unless under the direction of a physician.
2. Never use a coffee enema that is too hot. This can be painful and damaging. Like for real. Too cool is way better than too hot.
3. Never force the enema tip in.
4. Never force yourself to hold the enema longer than is comfortable.
5. Always lay on the right side instead of the left as you would typically do for a warm water enema.
6. Clean your enema bag often and be quick to replace equipment.

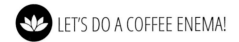 # LET'S DO A COFFEE ENEMA!

DIRECTIONS:

1. Put a little over 1 quart of purified water in a pan and bring it to a boil. Add 3 rounded tablespoons coffee. Continue to boil for five minutes. Turn the stove off.

2. Place coffee in a French press and allow to steep, until coffee is cooled to body temperature. If unsure, allow to cool more. It is safer to have the temperature too cool instead of too hot.

3. Lay an old towel on the bathroom floor. Bring a pillow or use additional towels to support your head. Bring relaxing reading materials.

4. If you have never used your enema bag, attach the enema attachment (not the douche attachment). Ensure that it is firmly attached.

5. Close the clamp on the enema hose. Pour the coffee into the enema bag avoiding adding coffee grounds. Do not use a paper filter to strain any remaining grounds. While holding enema tip over the sink, gently loosen the clamp and purge any air in the tubing by allowing a small amount of coffee to run through. Clamp again.

6. Hang the enema bag from a towel rack or another object at least 2 feet off the ground. Do not hang from a shower curtain rod.

7. Lie down on the floor on your right side and gently insert the catheter into your anus. Do not lay on the left side as this increases the risk of caffeine toxicity. If you need lubrication, any plant oil will work. KY Jelly is an alternative. I discourage you from using petrolatum products.

8. Gently insert the tube into the rectum a few inches and then release the clamp and let 2 cups of coffee flow in. Clamp the tubing off as soon as there is the slightest amount of discomfort or fullness.

9. Retain the enema for up to 12-15 minutes, or as long as you can hold it. If you feel the immediate need to go, that's okay. Never retain the enema for longer than is comfortable. Go to the toilet.

10. Repeat steps 8 and 9 to use the remaining 2 cups of water.

11. When finished, rinse the enema bag and tubing with hot water. Periodically clean enema bag and tubing with boiling water and hydrogen peroxide. Never use an enema bag as a douche bag.

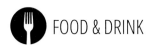 FOOD & DRINK

TODAY'S MENU

B: _____

L: _____

D: _____

REFLECTION ON THE DAY

HOW WAS YOUR SLEEP LAST NIGHT?

The worst, I barely slept   Like a rock

| 1 | 2 | 3 | 4 | 5 | 6 | 7 | 8 | 9 | 10 |

HOW IS YOUR ENERGY TODAY?

I am literally walking dead over here   I could probably run a marathon

| 1 | 2 | 3 | 4 | 5 | 6 | 7 | 8 | 9 | 10 |

THE QUALITY OF YOUR POOP THIS MORNING?

Smelly, severe constipation or diarrhea   Smooth, 10-12 inch masterpiece

| 1 | 2 | 3 | 4 | 5 | 6 | 7 | 8 | 9 | 10 |

HOW ARE YOUR FOOD CRAVINGS TODAY?

Somebody give me a doughnut now   What's to crave? This food is amazing!

| 1 | 2 | 3 | 4 | 5 | 6 | 7 | 8 | 9 | 10 |

REFLECTION ON TODAY

_____

_____

☐ CRUSHED IT!

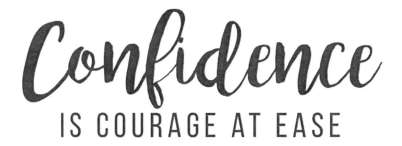

Confidence

IS COURAGE AT EASE

- D A N I E L   M A H E R -

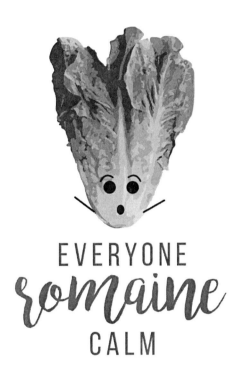

EVERYONE

romaine

CALM

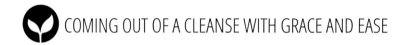

COMING OUT OF A CLEANSE WITH GRACE AND EASE

Coming out of a cleanse can be a double-edged sword. On the one hand, you may be ready to include some foods back into your diet. On the other, you may find that the foods you used to eat regularly are now too hard on your system. You may also find that if you introduce all of the foods at once, it is impossible to tell which ones are causing upset stomach, skin irritation, or allergies. For lack of a better word, I call the reintroduction phase the re-tox since we have spent 3 weeks going through a detox.

Over the next few days, I suggest that you take the reintroduction of each food very slowly. Please take at least five days to come out of the cleanse. Take each food component one at a time. For example, if you include gluten one day, do not also include caffeine or alcohol, even if you have tried them again following the cleanse.

If you choose to not reintroduce any foods, that is absolutely fine as well. There is no need to bring back any of the foods we eliminated from the cleanse, because, as we have seen for the past three weeks, there is no need to include any of them in your regular diet.

Today and tomorrow are a little bit different because, really, it is just 5 days-worth of exercise and reflection.

DAY 1: INTRODUCE CAFFEINE

I suggest a gentle form of caffeine such as that from green tea, and I advise against artificial caffeine, such as that found in many energy drinks and sodas, at any time on or off the cleanse. After you drink the tea, sit quietly for at least 15 minutes, preferably 30 minutes. In the following hours, continue to observe your heart rate, mental alertness, and breathing rate. Set an alarm to check these markers every 30 minutes to 1 hour for the next 8 hours. Set 15 minutes aside in the morning to write in your journal and consider how your sleep is the same or different than it was before.

DAY 2: INTRODUCE GLUTEN

No one is denying that gluten is exceptionally tasty, but it can wreak havoc on your gut and immune system. Pay attention to any underlying gastrointestinal disorders and autoimmune disorders for flare ups. The morning after eating gluten, be sure to observe the quality and consistency of your stool. Be sure to chew a lot as the gluten will be denser than most of the foods that we have been eating in the past few weeks.

DAY 3: INTRODUCE SUGAR

Or don't. Like for real. You really don't need sugar in your diet. However, I acknowledge that sweet treats can be so delicious on occasion. For this one I really want you to pay attention to how your mind feels after you eat as well as the food cravings that may arise in the hours after. Sugar has the potential to increase the desire for more sugar, so pay close attention.

DAY 4: INTRODUCE ALCOHOL

Take it easy here! Your tolerance has likely changed a lot since the beginning of the cleanse. Grab a glass of champagne or a spritzer before heading straight back to liquor. You may find that the morning after drinking hits you like a ton of bricks. Perhaps introduce alcohol on a day when you know that you are able to sleep in or have a quiet morning at home. After you have one drink, observe how you feel. How does your skin feel? Your heart rate? Your stomach? Pay attention to food cravings that may arise. Alcohol and the mixers that accompany them are generally packed full of sugar and can lead to blood sugar fluctuations. The next morning, be sure to assess your energy, sleep, and bowel movements. . . and even a potential headache.

DAY 5: INTRODUCE ANIMAL PRODUCTS

For me, the biggest changes in my body come whenever animal products are introduced. After I have been on a cleanse the first bite of cheese inevitably instantly causes mucous to form in my sinuses. Meat consistently slows down bowel movements in most people. I encourage you to bring forward a consciousness about meat into your everyday life. How was the animal raised? How was it slaughtered? What was it fed? This last point is critical because we are no longer bound by "You are what you eat". In the words of Michael Pollan, "You are what you eat eats". If you are consuming chicken that has eaten nothing but genetically modified corn intended to make the animal get fat fast, guess what may happen to you? I know for most people eating meat is almost a habit, and I encourage you to be aware of your actions as you eat.

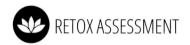 RETOX ASSESSMENT

ON EACH DAY OF YOUR RE-TOX ANSWER THE FOLLOWING QUESTIONS:

1. Describe how the food or beverage tastes on your palate.

2. Describe how your body feels in the 30 minutes after drinking/eating caffeine/eating gluten/sugar/ alcohol/animal product.

3. How does your body change in the hours after consumption of caffeine/gluten/sugar/alcohol animal product?

THE NEXT MORNING, ASSESS:

4. How is your energy level?

5. How was your sleep last night?

6. How was your poop this morning?

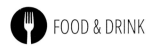 FOOD & DRINK

TODAY'S MENU

B: _____

L: _____

D: _____

REFLECTION ON THE DAY

HOW WAS YOUR SLEEP LAST NIGHT?

The worst, I barely slept   Like a rock

| 1 | 2 | 3 | 4 | 5 | 6 | 7 | 8 | 9 | 10 |

HOW IS YOUR ENERGY TODAY?

I am literally walking dead over here   I could probably run a marathon

| 1 | 2 | 3 | 4 | 5 | 6 | 7 | 8 | 9 | 10 |

THE QUALITY OF YOUR POOP THIS MORNING?

Smelly, severe constipation or diarrhea   Smooth, 10-12 inch masterpiece

| 1 | 2 | 3 | 4 | 5 | 6 | 7 | 8 | 9 | 10 |

HOW ARE YOUR FOOD CRAVINGS TODAY?

Somebody give me a doughnut now   What's to crave? This food is amazing!

| 1 | 2 | 3 | 4 | 5 | 6 | 7 | 8 | 9 | 10 |

REFLECTION ON TODAY

_____

_____

☐ CRUSHED IT!

A GREAT ACCOMPLISHMENT
SHOULDN'T BE THE END OF
THE ROAD, JUST THE
STARTING POINT FOR THE
next leap forward

- H A R V E Y M A C K A Y -

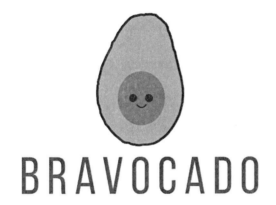

BRAVOCADO

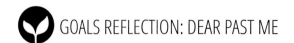 GOALS REFLECTION: DEAR PAST ME

So here we are! At the very end of our 21-day journey. Instead of looking at this as the end, I hope you will see this as a beginning to a lifestyle. You may choose to bring back in some of the forbidden foods, but I encourage you: do it with care. One thing is for sure, if you immediately go back to your previous way of eating, you will immediately slip back in to the habits that prompted you to start the cleanse in the first place. Think through why you originally started, your affirmations, and the positive statements that helped you to overcome opposition when you dined out. That strong, excellent version of you doesn't disappear simply because the cleanse is over. You honestly are likely a better version of yourself following the cleanse than you were before. I hope you come out of the cleanse with greater self-awareness, better cooking skills, and a greater love of food in general. I hope you come out of this loving yourself more.

To help you envision how your life may look following the cleanse, I have rewritten the Days -3-0 guidelines to be lifelong eating principles.

1. Bring your Friends and Family

   Nobody hates on a shared dish that is delicious. Bring food and share freely. Don't even mention that it is vegan. Just share.

2. Bring along Convenience Foods

   Always. Pack. Snacks.

3. Keep the Pantry Clean

   The less crap you have in your home, the less crap you eat.

4. Add New Ingredients to Compliment the Staples

   Embrace the opportunity to eat new foods. Farmers market ugly vegetables for the win.

5. Master Nextovers

   Make it a bowl, salad, or pasta.

6. Shop with Ease

   For my shopping suggestions come to www.amazon.com/shop/lindseyelmore

7. Dine Out with Care

   Man, oh man, can dining out change your palate. Choose the healthiest options available.

8. Strategically Grocery Shop

   Plan meals and make life easy.

9. Discover New Recipes

   Get your Pinterest on.

10. Embrace the Success and Struggle

    Life ain't always easy. Do your best. Forget the Rest.

Today we are actually going to do two exercises to end our cleanse. First, let's review our goals from the beginning of the cleanse. Flip back to Day 1 and see how far you have come. You are a different person now. I am proud of you. And even if no one else tells you today, I love you. Remember that. You are deeply loved. You are valued. You are you. And what a miracle that is.

1. List 3 reasons you are grateful you did this cleanse.

_____

_____

_____

2. What was the best thing that happened during the cleanse?

_____

3. What did you accomplish in the past 21 days?

_____

4. What do you most appreciate?

_____

5. What do you most regret?

_____

6. What challenges did you meet?

_____

_____

7. What did you do when challenges arose?

_____

8. List your 3 new favorite foods.

_____

_____

_____

9. List your 3 favorite vegan recipes.

_____

_____

_____

10. List 3 questions you know how to answer about vegan cleanses. Write down the answers.

_____

_____

_____

11. What did you most want to see at the beginning of the cleanse? Do you see it? If not, what other positive changes do you see?

_____

_____

_____

12. What did you learn on the cleanse that you will bring forward into your everyday life?

_____

13. At the end of this 21-day cleanse, I am. . .

_____

_____

_____

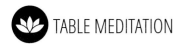 TABLE MEDITATION

This is another adapted meditation from Chel Hamilton on the Meditation Minis podcast.[1] You can watch me lead meditations on my YouTube Channel: https://bit.ly/2t4p7qj.

INSTRUCTIONS FOR MEDITATION

1. Come to a comfortable seated position.
2. Invite your eyes to close, take 3 deep breaths, and allow yourself to relax.
3. I want you to allow your mind to drift back to the weeks before the cleanse. I want you to think of everything you ate and drank in the weeks leading up to the cleanse. Picture it on a table in front of you. Be sure to keep everything in mind: breakfast, lunch, dinner, snacks, and drinks.
4. In your mind's eye, turn now to the other side of the room. See another banquet table laid out with everything you have eaten during the cleanse. All the fruits, vegetables, water, and new foods you had never tried before.
5. Now, I want you to turn back to the table that contains the foods you ate before the cleanse started. On that table, find the foods that are approved for the cleanse, and go grab them. Bring them over to your cleanse table.
6. All of a sudden, you start to notice a smell. A stench that you can't quite place. You turn back to the table of food from before the cleanse and notice that some of the foods have started to rot. Thankfully, you glance to the right and notice a rubbish bin.
7. You grab the bin and start to throw away all of the food left on the table from before the cleanse. Once it is full, you are able to take it out of the room.
8. You come back into the banquet hall, and the only food left is the food from the cleanse. Bright, vibrant, delicious food that serves your body well.
9. As you come out of the cleanse, remember the difference between the two tables. Remember how they looked in your mind's eye and remind yourself how your body feels when you eat from one table versus the other. Are you bringing in rotten food or fresh vibrant energy into your body?
10. Take three final cleansing breaths and whenever you are ready, open your eyes.

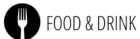 FOOD & DRINK

TODAY'S MENU

B: _____

L: _____

D: _____

REFLECTION ON THE DAY

HOW WAS YOUR SLEEP LAST NIGHT?

The worst, I barely slept   Like a rock

1   2   3   4   5   6   7   8   9   10

HOW IS YOUR ENERGY TODAY?

I am literally walking dead over here   I could probably run a marathon

1   2   3   4   5   6   7   8   9   10

THE QUALITY OF YOUR POOP THIS MORNING?

Smelly, severe constipation or diarrhea   Smooth, 10-12 inch masterpiece

1   2   3   4   5   6   7   8   9   10

HOW ARE YOUR FOOD CRAVINGS TODAY?

Somebody give me a doughnut now   What's to crave? This food is amazing!

1   2   3   4   5   6   7   8   9   10

REFLECTION ON TODAY

_____

_____

☐ CRUSHED IT!

APPENDICES

APPENDIX 1

Cleaning out the pantry of all the food that you will not be consuming in the next couple of weeks is a quick and easy way to stay on track. Below is a list of ingredients that you can bring into your pantry that will be used over and over again.

PANTRY LIST

ITEM	NOTES
BAKING GOODS AND FLOURS	
Agave nectar	
Almond Flour	
Arrowroot Powder	
Baking Powder	
Chickpea Flour	
Coconut Flour	
Gluten-Free Flour	
Oat Flour	
Tapioca Starch	
Vanilla Extract	
DRY GOODS	
Bread Crumbs	Gluten-Free
Chickpeas	Canned
Coconut	Shredded, Flaked
Dijon Mustard	

ITEM	NOTES
Herbal Tea	Mint, Chamomile, Vanilla Spice, Etc.
Hoisin Sauce	
Hot Sauce (optional)	
Lemon Juice	
Liquid Aminos	
Mustard	
Non-Dairy Protein Powder	
Oats	Old-Fashioned, Steel Cut, Quick
Pasta	Gluten-Free
Quinoa	
Rice	Brown, Jasmine
Salsa	Sugar-Free
Soy Sauce	Gluten-Free
Sriracha Sauce	
Stevia	
Tahini	Unsweetened
Tamari	
Vegetarian Stock	Better than Bullion
Vinegars	Apple Cider, Balsamic, Red Wine, Rice
Xylitol	

ITEM	NOTES
NUTS, SEEDS, NUT BUTTERS	
Almond Butter	Unsweetened
Almonds	
Cashew Butter	Unsweetened
Cashews	
Chia Seeds	
Flax Seeds	
Hemp Seeds	
Macadamia Nuts	
Peanut Butter	Unsweetened
Peanuts	
Pepitas (Pumpkin Seeds)	
Sesame Seeds	
Sunflower Seeds	
Walnuts	
COOKING OILS	
Avocado	
Canola	Expeller-Pressed Organic Non-GMO
Coconut	
Flax Seed	

ITEM	NOTES
Grapeseed	
Olive	Extra-Virgin
Safflower	High-Oleic
Sesame	
Sunflower	High-Oleic
Walnut	
REFRIGERATED	
Hummus	Plain or Flavored
Vegan Butter	Earth Balance
Vegan Salad Dressing	Tessamae's
Vegan Sour Cream	
SNACKS	
Crackers	Gluten-Free
Popcorn	Non-GMO
SPICES AND SEASONINGS	
Allspice	
Basil	Dried
Bay Leaves	
Berebere Spice	
Cayenne Pepper	

ITEM	NOTES
Celery Seed	Or Celery Seed Essential Oil
Chili Powder	
Cinnamon	Ground
Coriander	
Cumin Powder	
Curry Powder	
Dill	Dried, Or Dill Essential Oil
Garlic Powder	
Garlic Salt	
Ginger	Ground
Nutmeg	
Nutritional Yeast	
Onion Powder	
Oregano	Dried
Paprika	
Pepper	
Red Pepper Flakes	
Rosemary	
Salt	Pink Himalayan
Sea salt	
Turmeric Powder	

APPENDIX 2

Grocery Lists for Meal Plan (see pp. 22 – 25)

These grocery lists are designed to be your shopping lists if you decide to eat everything on the suggested menu. Before you shop, be sure to check your pantry items so you don't over purchase. For example, rice is needed each week of the cleanse, but you will likely not need a new bag each week.

WEEK 1 GROCERY LIST

ITEM	QUANTITY NEEDED	DAY(S) NEEDED
REFRIGERATED AND FROZEN ITEMS		
Almond Milk	1 Carton	1, 5, 7
Frozen Blueberries	2 Cups	2
Hummus	1 Small Container	1
Tofu, Extra Firm (16 oz.)	4 Blocks	1, 2, 3, 6
Tofu, Silken (16 oz.)	1 Block	6
Vegan Butter	1 Container	1, 2, 5, 7
Vegan Cheese, Grated (Optional)	½ Cup	6
Vegan Sour Cream (Optional)	1 Container	6
NUTS AND GRAINS		
Almonds, Raw and Unsalted	½ Cup	7
Brown Rice	2 Cups	1
Cashews, Raw and Unsalted	1 Cup	6, 7
Chia Seeds	6 Tablespoons	1
Flour, Chick Pea	2 Cups	5

ITEM	QUANTITY NEEDED	DAY(S) NEEDED
Flour, Gluten-Free	¼ Cup	5
Flour, Oat	1 Cup	2
Green Lentils	1½ Cups	6
Hemp Seeds	6 Tablespoons	6, 7
Old Fashioned Oats	1 Cup	2
Peanuts	½ Cup	1, 3
Pecan Halves	1¼ Cups	7
Pepitas (Pumpkin Seeds)	1 Small Container	7
Pine Nuts	¼ Cup	2
Rice, Jasmine	2 Cups	2, 3
Sesame Seeds (Optional)	1 Small Container	3
Tahini	1 Bottle or Jar	6
Walnuts	2 Tablespoons	2
FRESH HERBS		
Basil	2 bunches	4, 6
Cilantro	2 Bunches	1, 3, 4
Parsley, Flat Leaf	2 Bunches	1, 2, 4, 5, 6, 7
Tarragon Leaves	1 bunch	6
Thyme	1 bunch	4, 5, 6

ITEM	QUANTITY NEEDED	DAY(S) NEEDED
FRUITS		
Apples	2 Medium	5
Apples, Granny Smith	2 Medium	1, 3
Bananas	5 Medium	2, 7
Blackberries (optional)	1 Container	1
Lemons	5	1, 5, 6, 7
Limes	4	1, 2, 4, 5
Orange	1	3
Pear	1	5
Red Grapes	1 Cup	7
VEGETABLES		
Baby Bok Choy	6 Heads	1
Beets, Golden	1 Medium	3
Broccoli	2 Heads	7
Brussels Sprouts	1 Pound	7
Cabbage, Red (Optional)	1 Small Head	3, 5
Carrots	1 Large Bag	3, 5, 6, 7
Celery	1 Head	1, 6, 7
Cucumber	1 Large	1
Eggplant	2 Medium	4

ITEM	QUANTITY NEEDED	DAY(S) NEEDED
Garlic Cloves	2 Bulbs	Multiple
Ginger	1 Small Knob	1, 3
Kaffir Lime Leaves	6 Leaves	2
Kale	6 Large	1, 6
Leeks	2 Medium	5
Lemongrass	1 Stalk	2
Mushrooms, Baby Bella	8 oz.	3
Mushrooms, Cremini	5 oz.	5
Mushrooms, Portobello	5 Ounces	5
Mushrooms, Shiitake	2 Cups	1, 5
Onions, Green	2 Bunches	1, 2, 3, 5
Onions, Yellow	6 Medium	2, 3, 4, 5, 6, 7
Peppers, Green Bell	1 Small	6
Peppers, Jalapeño	1 Medium	4
Peppers, Yellow Bell	1 Large	4
Peppers, Red Bell	3 Small	2, 4, 6
Potatoes, Baby Gold	2 Pounds	6
Radishes	2 Medium	6
Romaine Lettuce	4 Heads	3, 6
Shallots	2 Medium	7

ITEM	QUANTITY NEEDED	DAY(S) NEEDED
Spring Mix Salad Greens	1 Medium Container	2, 3
Squash, Butternut	1 Large	7
Squash, Yellow	2 Medium	4
Squash, Zucchini	3 To 4 Medium	4, 7
Sweet Potatoes	1 Medium	1
Thai Chilies	3	2
Tomatoes, Cherry or Grape	1 pint	1, 6
Tomatoes, Roma	6 Medium	4
Turmeric	3 Thumb Size Knobs	3
PANTRY INGREDIENTS		
Agave Nectar	1 Bottle	1
Apple Cider Vinegar	1 Bottle	6
Balsamic Vinegar	1 Medium Bottle	Multiple
Capers	1 Jar	6, 7
Chickpeas (15 oz.)	2 – 14 oz. cans	1, 6
Coconut Milk (15 oz.)	2 – 15 oz. Can	2, 7
Corn (15 oz.)	1 – 14 oz. Can	5
Crushed Tomatoes (15 oz.)	1 – 28 oz. Can	4
Diced Canned Tomatoes (15 oz.)	1 – 14 oz. Can	6
Dijon Mustard	1 Bottle	6

ITEM	QUANTITY NEEDED	DAY(S) NEEDED
Hoisin Sauce	1 Bottle	3
Liquid Aminos	1 Bottle	2
Oil, Coconut	1 Medium Jar	1, 2
Oil, Grapeseed	1 Bottle	1, 3
Oil, Olive	1 Small Bottle	Multiple
Oil, Sesame	1 Small Bottle	3
Rice Vinegar	1 Bottle	1, 3, 6
Salsa (Optional)	1 Medium Container	6
Tamari	1 Bottle	1, 3
Thai Green Curry Paste	1 Small Container	2
Vegetable Stock or Base	4 Cartons or 1 Jar Base	1, 4, 5, 6, 7
Water Chestnuts (8 oz.)	1 Can	3
DRY SPICES		
Bay Leaves	1 Jar	6
Cayenne Pepper	1 Small Jar	6
Chili Powder	1 Small Jar	3, 6
Cinnamon, Ground	1 Small Jar	7
Cumin	1 Small Jar	6
Dried Dill, or Dill Essential Oil	1 Jar or 1 Bottle	1
Garlic Powder	1 Small Jar	6, 7

ITEM	QUANTITY NEEDED	DAY(S) NEEDED
Nutritional Yeast	1 Medium Jar	5, 6, 7
Oregano, Dried	1 Small Jar	7
Red Pepper Flakes	1 Small Jar	3
Turmeric Powder	1 Small Jar	6

WEEK 2 GROCERY LIST

ITEM	QUANTITY NEEDED	DAY(S) NEEDED
REFRIGERATED AND FROZEN ITEMS		
Almond Milk	1 Carton	9, 12
Guacamole (Optional)	1 Tub	14
Tempeh	1 Block	10
Tofu, Extra Firm (16 oz.)	4 Blocks	8, 13, 14
Vegan Butter	1 Small Container	Multiple
Vegan Cheese, Grated	5 Cups	12, 13, 14
Vegan Mayonnaise	1 Jar	8
Vegan Ricotta	¾ Cup	11
Vegan Sour Cream (Optional)	1 Container	13, 14
NUTS AND GRAINS		
Almonds, Raw and Unsalted	1 ½ Cups	10, 11
Arrowroot Powder	3 Tablespoons	14
Cashews, Raw and Unsalted	2 Cups	8, 10, 11, 14
Chia Seeds	¼ Cup	9
Coconut, Shredded	½ Cup	10
Flax Seeds, Ground	6 Tablespoons	12, 13
Flour, Almond	½ Cup	13
Flour, Chick Pea	1 Cup	11

ITEM	QUANTITY NEEDED	DAY(S) NEEDED
Flour, Oat	2 Cups	12
Hemp Seeds	⅓ Cup	9, 12, 14
Lentils, Green	1½ Cups (Cooked)	8
Lentils, Sprouted Green	½ Cup	9
Macadamia Nuts, Raw and Unsalted	½ Cup	11
Oats, Steel Cut	1 Cup	8
Peanut Butter, Crunchy	¼ Cup	14
Peanuts, Raw and Unsalted	1 Jar	14
Pecan Halves, Raw and Unsalted	½ Cup	11
Rice, Black	1 Cup	10
Rice, Jasmine	2 Cups	13
Sesame Seeds, Black	1 Teaspoon	14
Tahini	1 Jar	8, 9
Tapioca Starch	1 Tablespoon	10
Walnuts, Raw and Unsalted	1½ Cups	10, 11
DRY SPICES		
Basil	1 Bunch	14
Cilantro	1 Bunch	10, 14
Mint	1 Bunch	9, 14
Parsley, Curly	1 Bunch	9

ITEM	QUANTITY NEEDED	DAY(S) NEEDED
Parsley, Flat Leaf	1 Bunch	8, 12
Rosemary	1 Bunch	12
Thyme	1 Bunch	11, 14
FRUITS		
Apples, Granny Smith	5	9, 10, 11
Avocado	2	9
Bananas	3	9, 11
Berries	2-3 Pints	8, 9, 11
Figs	3	11
Lemons	6	Multiple
Limes	2	10
Orange	1	11
VEGETABLES		
Arugula	2 Cups	11
Beets, Golden	2	12
Beets, Red	4	11, 12
Bok Choy	6 Small Heads	14
Broccoli	1 Head	13
Cabbage, Red	1	10
Carrots	1 lb. Bag	10, 11, 14

ITEM	QUANTITY NEEDED	DAY(S) NEEDED
Celery	1 Small Bunch	9
Cucumber	3	9, 14
Eggplant	2	12
Fennel Bulb	2	9, 11
Garlic Cloves	2 Bulbs	Multiple
Ginger	1-2 Large Chunk	Multiple
Kale	1 Bunch	9
Kale, Lacinato	5 Stems	10
Leeks	3	11
Lemongrass	1	9
Lettuce, Red Leaf	12 Leaves	14
Lettuce, Romaine	1 Bunch	8
Mung Bean Sprouts	1 Cup	14
Mushrooms, Baby Bella	2 ½ Cups	8
Onions, Green	1 To 2 Bunch	9, 14
Onions, Red	1	8
Onions, Spanish	1	14
Onions, White	4	11, 13
Onions, Yellow	5	Multiple
Parsnips	3 Medium	12

ITEM	QUANTITY NEEDED	DAY(S) NEEDED
Peppers, Red Bell	2	10, 13
Peppers, Yellow Bell	1	13
Potatoes	4 Medium	13
Rutabaga	1 Medium	12
Snap Peas	Handful	10
Spinach	1 lb.	12
Squash, Spaghetti	1	9
Tomatoes, Grape	1 Pint	9
PANTRY		
Agave Nectar	1 Bottle	Multiple
Applesauce (Optional)	1 Jar	13
Beans, Refried Pinto, Vegetarian (15 oz.)	1 Can	14
Bread Crumbs, Gluten-Free	2 ½ Cups	12
Chickpeas (15 oz.)	6 Cans	12
Coconut Milk (15 oz.)	3 Cans	9, 10, 11
Corn (15 oz.)	1 Can	14
Corn Tortillas	10 To 12	14
Crackers, Gluten-Free	1 Package	12
Dill Pickles	Small Jar	8
Hamburger Buns, Gluten-Free	1 Package	8

ITEM	QUANTITY NEEDED	DAY(S) NEEDED
Jicama	1 Jar	9
Oil, Avocado	1 Bottle	14
Oil, Canola	1 Small Bottle	9, 14
Oil, Coconut	1 Jar	Multiple
Oil, Olive	1 Bottle	Multiple
Oil, Peanut	1 Bottle	14
Oil, Sesame	1 Bottle	14
Oil, Truffle (Optional)	1 Bottle	12
Pasta, Gluten-Free	1 Box	14
Pumpkin Puree (15 oz.)	1 Can	12
Raisins, Golden	1 Small Package	11
Rice Noodles	2 oz.	14
Rice Spring Roll Wrappers	1 Package	14
Roasted Red Peppers	1 Jar	9
Salsa (Optional)	1 Jar	14
Sriracha Sauce (Optional)	1 Bottle	14
Tamari	1 Bottle	14
Tomato Paste (4 oz.)	1 Can	14
Tomatoes, Whole Peeled (15 oz.)	2 Cans	14
Vanilla Extract	1 bottle	9, 12

ITEM	QUANTITY NEEDED	DAY(S) NEEDED
Vegetable Stock	2 – 32 oz. cartons	9, 11, 14
Vinegar, Rice Wine	1 Bottle	10, 14
Wraps, Gluten-Free (Optional)	1 Package	8
DRY SPICES		
Celery Seed	1 Small Jar	8
Chili Flakes	1 Jar	10, 14
Chili Powder	1 Jar	Multiple
Cinnamon, Ground	1 Jar	Multiple
Cumin	1 Jar	14
Curry Powder	1 Small Jar	8
Garlic Powder	1 Jar	9, 14
German Mustard	1 Jar	14
Ginger, Ground	1 Small Jar	9, 12
Green Curry Paste	1 Small Jar	10
Lavender Buds	2 TBSP	13
Nutmeg, Ground	1 Small Jar	12
Nutritional Yeast	1 Medium Container	8, 12, 14
Onion Powder	1 Jar	14
Oregano, Dried	1 Jar	14
Paprika, Smoked	1 Small Bottle	8
Turmeric Powder	1 Small Jar	8, 9, 11, 14

WEEK 3 GROCERY LIST

ITEM	QUANTITY NEEDED	DAY(S) NEEDED
REFRIGERATED AND FROZEN ITEMS		
Almond Milk	1 Carton	17, 18, 19, 20, 21
Guacamole (Optional)	1 Tub	18
Peaches (May Use Fresh)	3 Pounds	18
Tofu, Silken (16 oz.)	3 Blocks	19, 20, 21
Vegan Butter	1 Small Container	17, 21
Vegan Cheese, Grated	1 Cup	16, 19
Vegan Sour Cream	1 Container	15, 16, 17
Young Jackfruit	2 Pouches	16
NUTS AND GRAINS		
Almonds, Raw and Unsalted	⅔ Cup	18
Arrowroot Starch or Corn Starch	1 Tablespoon	16
Cashews, Raw and Unsalted	3 Cups	15, 16, 19, 20
Chia Seeds	¼ Cup	17
Coconut, Flakes	2 Tablespoons	18
Flax Seed Meal, Golden	1 Tablespoon	19
Flax Seeds, Ground	2 Teaspoons	21
Flour, Chick Pea	1 ¼ Cup	16, 21
Flour, Coconut	2 Teaspoons	18

ITEM	QUANTITY NEEDED	DAY(S) NEEDED
Flour, Gluten-Free	1 Teaspoon	20
Flour, Tapioca	1 Cup	19
Hemp Seeds	2 Tablespoons	19
Oats, Quick	½ Cup	21
Oats, Steel Cut	¾ Cup	19
Peanut Butter	1 Tablespoon	19
Peanuts, Raw and Unsalted	¾ Cup	18
Pecan Halves, Raw and Unsalted	⅔ Cup	18
Pecans, Chopped	1 Cup	19, 20
Pine Nuts	¼ Cup	16
Potato Starch	½ Cup	19
Pepitas (Pumpkin Seeds) (Optional)	½ Cup	17
Quinoa	1 Cup	16
Rice, Brown	1 Cup	18
FRESH HERBS		
Basil	1 Bunch	19, 21
Cilantro	2 Bunches	16, 17, 18, 21
Dill	1 Bunch	15, 19
Mint	1 Bunch	14, 15
Parsley, Flat Leaf	1 Bunch	15, 18, 19

ITEM	QUANTITY NEEDED	DAY(S) NEEDED
Thyme	1 Bunch	16
FRUIT		
Apple, Granny Smith	1	15
Avocado	3	16, 17, 21
Bananas	4	19, 21
Blackberries	2 Cups	18
Blueberries	1 Cup	18
Cranberries	1 Cup	21
Dates	4	18
Lemons	4	Multiple
Limes	3	16, 17, 18, 21
Orange	1	21
Peaches (May Use Frozen)	3 Pounds	18
VEGETABLES		
Asparagus	20 Spears	17
Beets, Red	3 Medium	15
Broccoli	9 Cups	19, 20
Cabbage, Red	1 Head	15, 16
Carrots	1 lb. Bag	15, 17, 18, 20
Cauliflower	4 Heads	16, 17, 18, 21

ITEM	QUANTITY NEEDED	DAY(S) NEEDED
Celery	1 Bunch	15, 17, 18, 20
Collard Greens	1 Head	17
Cucumber	2	15, 17, 19
Garlic	1-2 Heads	Multiple
Ginger	Thumb Size	18
Jalapeño	2	17, 18
Kale, Baby	1 Cup	16
Kale, Lacinato	1 Bunch	20
Lettuce, Iceburg (Optional)	1 Head	16
Lettuce, Romaine	2 Bunch	15, 21
Onions, Green	1 Bunch	16
Onions, Red	3	16, 19, 20
Onions, White	2	16, 20
Onions, Yellow	6	Multiple
Parsnips	2 Large	17
Pepper, Green Bell	1	17
Potatoes, Russett	1 Medium	15
Potatoes, Yellow	5	15, 20
Shallot	1	17
Spinach	¾ Cup	19

ITEM	QUANTITY NEEDED	DAY(S) NEEDED
Squash, Butternut	1	16
Sweet Potatoes	1 Large	20
Tomatoes	4	16, 18, 19
Tomatoes, Grape or Cherry	1 Pint	16, 21
PANTRY ITEMS		
Agave Nectar	1 Bottle	Multiple
Beans, Black (15 oz.)	1 Can	18
Beans, Pinto, Vegetarian (15 oz.)	1 Can	16
Beans, Refried Pinto, Vegetarian (15 oz.)	1 Can	21
Bread Crumbs, Gluten-Free	1 Container	15
Capers	1 Jar	17
Chickpeas (15 oz.)	1 Can	17
Club Soda	1 Bottle	17, 21
Coconut Cream	1 Can	18
Corn (15 oz.) (Optional)	1 Can	18
Corn Tortillas	20 Tortillas	16, 21
Hot Sauce	1 Small Jar	19, 21
Jackfruit	2 Pouches or Cans	16
Macaroni Noodles, Gluten-Free	1 Package	15
Mustard (Optional)	1 Jar	16, 20

ITEM	QUANTITY NEEDED	DAY(S) NEEDED
Oil, Canola	1 Bottle	18
Oil, Coconut	1 Jar	16, 18, 19
Oil, Grapeseed	1 Bottle	16
Oil, Olive	1 Bottle	Multiple
Oil, Sesame	1 Bottle	18
Pumpkin Puree (15 oz.)	1 Can	17
Raisins	1 Package	20
Salsa (Optional)	1 Jar	16
Sriracha Sauce (Optional)	1 Bottle	16, 18
Tomato Juice (Sugar-Free)	1 Jar	19
Tomato Paste (4 oz.)	1 Can	15
Tomatoes w/ Green Chilies, Chopped (15 oz.)	1 Can	18
Vanilla Extract	1 Bottle	17
Vegetable Stock	4 Boxes	15, 16, 18, 19, 20
Vinegar, Apple Cider	1 Bottle	16, 20
Vinegar, Red Wine	1 Bottle	18, 19
Vinegar, Rice Wine	1 Bottle	18
Vinegar, White Wine	1 Bottle	16, 21
Worcestershire Sauce	1 Bottle	19

ITEM	QUANTITY NEEDED	DAY(S) NEEDED
DRY SPICES		
Allspice	1 Jar	18
Bay Leaves	1 Jar	20
Berebere Spice	1 Jar	20
Cayenne Pepper, Ground	1 Jar	16, 18, 20
Celery Salt	1 Jar	19
Celery Seed (Optional)	1 Jar	20
Chili Flakes	1 Jar	18
Chili Pepper, Chipotle (Optional)	1 Jar	20
Chili Powder	1 Jar	16
Chives, Dried	1 Jar	19, 21
Cinnamon, Ground	1 Jar	18, 19
Coriander	1 Jar	16, 18
Cumin	1 Jar	16, 18
Dill Seed (Optional)	1 Jar	20
Dill, Dried	1 Jar	19, 21
Garlic Powder	1 Jar	16, 19, 21
Ginger, Ground	1 Jar	18
Herbs de Provence	1 Jar	17
Mustard, Dry	1 Jar	17

ITEM	QUANTITY NEEDED	DAY(S) NEEDED
Nutritional Yeast	1 Jar	19, 21
Onion Powder	1 Jar	16, 20
Onion, Dried Minced	1 Jar	19, 21
Oregano, Dried	1 Jar	16, 18
Paprika	1 Jar	16, 18, 21
Parsley, Dried	1 Jar	19, 21
Pumpkin Pie Spice	1 Jar	17
Turmeric	1 Jar	21

APPENDIX 3 - READ, WATCH, AND LISTEN

Below is a list of books, films and mini-series that I love to watch about food, food politics, the ability of food to heal common ailments, and the overall power of food to be a transformative force in your life. Some are challenging to take in, others are outside of the scope of this cleanse, but I have read or watched them all. They have influenced my opinions on food and created the version of eating that courses through my everyday life. For links to purchase, head to https://www.amazon.com/shop/lindseyelmore.

BOOKS ABOUT FOOD

The China Study, T. Colin and Thomas Campbell

In Defense of Food, Michael Pollan

The Omnivore's Dilemma, Michael Pollan

Women, Food and God, Geneen Roth

Quantum Wellness, Kathy Freston

Fast Food Nation, Eric Schlosser

Animal, Vegetable, Miracle, Barbara Kingsolver

Salt: A World History, Mark Kurlansky

FOOD DOCUMENTARIES

What the Health

Forks Over Knives

Food, Inc.

Cowspiracy

Rotten

Fat, Sick and Nearly Dead

Super Size Me

Dying to Have Known

The Beautiful Truth

The Gerson Miracle

Wasted

Fed Up

Hungry for Change

FOOD DOCU-SERIES

Cooked

Rotten

Wasted!

APPENDIX 4 - RECOMMENDED BRANDS

Since my house is consistently gluten-free and vegan, I have a lot of experience testing different ingredients. Below is a list of my favorite brands and ingredients. For links to these and many more of my favorite products, head over to https://www.amazon.com/shop/lindseyelmore

BANZA CHICKPEA PASTA: Hands down the best gluten-free, Italian style noodle out there. I don't love it for Asian dishes, but for any Italian or American dish, this is my go-to noodle.

BETTER THAN BULLION VEGETABLE BASE: the most amazing, nearly instant stock is at your disposal.

BEYOND BURGER AND SAUSAGES: You will never miss ground beef or pork with these absolutely delicious burgers and sausages.

DAIRY FREE CHEESES AND CREAMS: Chao, Follow Your Heart Vegan Parmesan, Kite Hill, Daiya Cream Cheese, Tofutti Sour Cream

ITHACA HUMMUS: The Fresh Lemon Dill is one of my favorites, but I also love the classic, Lemon Garlic, Lemon Beet, and more.

GLUTINO PRETZELS: Literally better than gluten-filled pretzels.

PURPLE CARROT'S TBL MEALS: gluten-free, vegan food delivery boxes? Yes, please!

SCHAR GLUTEN-FREE BREAD: I know, I know. I am breaking my own rules by including this product because it contains a tiny bit of honey, but it is the only gluten-free bread I have found that does not contain egg. Pick your battles.

VEGAN ROBS: Cheddar Puffs, Brussel Sprout Puffs, and Cauliflower puffs. I swear the cheddar puffs are better than the original without all the weird coloring agents.

XOCHITL CORN CHIPS: Although they are annoyingly thin when eating dips, these are the best corn chips I have ever tasted.

REFERENCES

THREE DAYS BEFORE YOU CLEANSE

1. Duhigg C. The Power of Habit: Why We Do What We Do in Life and Business. 2014. Random House Trade Paperbacks.

DAY 1: WHY CLEANSE?

1. Callahan E. Changes in weight loss and lipid profiles after a dietary purification program: a prospective case series. J Chiropr Med. 2013 Mar;12(1):30-8. doi: 10.1016/j.jcm.2012.11.004.
2. Balliett M, Burke JR. Changes in anthropometric measurements, body composition, blood pressure, lipid profile, and testosterone in patients participating in a low-energy dietary intervention. J Chiropr Med. 2013 Mar;12(1):3-14. doi: 10.1016/j.jcm.2012.11.003.
3. Ho CP, Yu JH, Lee TJF. Ovo-vegetarian diet is associated with lower systemic blood pressure in Taiwanese women. Public Health. 2017 Sep 25;153:70-77. doi: 10.1016/j.puhe.2017.07.032. [Epub ahead of print].
4. Kahleova H, Levin S, Barnard N. Cardio-Metabolic Benefits of Plant-Based Diets. Nutrients. 2017;9(8):848. doi:10.3390/nu9080848.

DAY 2: WHY AVOID CAFFEINE?

1. Gilbert RM. Caffeine consumption. In: The Methylxanthine Beverages and Foods: Chemistry, Consumption, and Health Effects. G.A. Spiller (Ed). New York: Alan R. Liss, Inc.;1984: pp. 185–213.
2. Frary CD, Johnson RK, Wang MQ. Food sources and intakes of caffeine in the diets of persons in the United States. J Am Diet Assoc. 2005; 105:110–113.
3. Higdon JV, Frei B. Coffee and health: a review of recent human research. Crit Rev Food Sci Nutr. 2006;46:101–123.
4. Nawrot P, Jordan S, Eastwood J, Rotstein J, Hugenholtz A, Feeley M. Effects of caffeine on human health. Food Addit Contam. 2003;20:1–30.
5. Rhee J, Kim R, Kim Y, et al. Maternal Caffeine Consumption during Pregnancy and Risk of Low Birth Weight: A Dose-Response Meta-Analysis of Observational Studies. Zhang B, ed. PLoS ONE. 2015;10(7):e0132334. doi:10.1371/journal.pone.0132334.
6. Katan MB, Schouten E. Caffeine and arrhythmia. Am J Clin Nutr March 2005 vol. 81 no. 3 539-540.
7. Higgins JP, Yarlagadda S and Yang B Cardiovascular Complications of Energy Drinks Beverages 2015, 1, 104-126; doi:10.3390/beverages1020104
8. Conti CR, Clinical Cardiology Volume 14, Issue 2, Version of Record online: 4 FEB 2009.
9. Solinas M, Ferre S, You ZB, Karcz-Kubicha M, Popoli P, Goldberg SR. Caffeine induces dopamine and glutamate release in the shell of the nucleus accumbens. J Neurosci. 2002;22:6321–6324.
10. Pontieri FE, Tanda G, Di Chiara G. Intravenous cocaine, morphine, and amphetamine preferentially increase extracellular dopamine in the "shell" as compared with the "core" of the rat nucleus accumbens. Proc Natl Acad Sci USA. 1995;92:12304–12308.

11. Wise RA, Bozarth MA. A psychomotor stimulant theory of addiction. Psychol Rev. 1987;94:469–492.

12. Borycz J, Pereira MF, Melani A, Rodrigues RJ, Kofalvi A, Panlilio L, et al. Differential glutamate-dependent and glutamate-independent adenosine A1 receptor-mediated modulation of dopamine release in different striatal compartments. J Neurochem. 2007;101:355–363.

13. Quarta D, Borycz J, Solinas M, Patkar K, Hockemeyer J, Ciruela F, et al, Adenosine receptor-mediated modulation of dopamine release in the nucleus accumbens depends on glutamate neurotransmission and N-methyl-D-aspartate receptor stimulation. J Neurochem. 2004;91:873–880.

14. Quarta D, Ferre S, Solinas M, You ZB, Hockemeyer J, Popoli P, et al. Opposite modulatory roles for adenosine A1 and A2A receptors on glutamate and dopamine release in the shell of the nucleus accumbens. Effects of chronic caffeine exposure. J Neurochem. 2004;88:1151–1158.

15. How does caffeine affect the body? Scientific American. Available at: https://www.scientificamerican.com/article/how-does-caffeine-affect/. Last accessed January 25, 2019.

16. Yamada Y, Nakazato Y, Ohga A. The mode of action of caffeine on catecholamine release from perfused adrenal glands of cat. British Journal of Pharmacology. 1989;98(2):351-356.

17. Begas E, Kouvaras E, Tsakalof A, Papakosta S, Asprodini E K in Biomedical chromatography : BMC (2007). In vivo evaluation of CYP1A2, CYP2A6, NAT-2 and xanthine oxidase activities in a Greek population sample by the RP-HPLC monitoring of caffeine metabolic ratios by the RP-HPLC monitoring of caffeine metabolic ratios.

18. Juliano LM, Huntley ED, Harrell PT, Westerman AT. Development of the caffeine withdrawal symptom questionnaire: caffeine withdrawal symptoms cluster into 7 factors. Drug Alcohol Depend. 2012;124:229–234.

19. Juliano LM, Griffiths RR. A critical review of caffeine withdrawal: empirical validation of symptoms and signs, incidence, severity, and associated features. Psychopharmacology (Berl). 2004;176:1–29.

20. Evans SM, Griffiths RR. Caffeine withdrawal: a parametric analysis of caffeine dosing conditions. J Pharmacol Exp Ther. 1999;289:285–294.

ADDITIONAL REFERENCES RELATED TO CAFFEINE DEPENDENCE

21. Anderson BL, Juliano LM. Behavior, sleep, and problematic caffeine consumption in a college-aged sample. J Caffeine Res. 2012;2:38–44.

22. Bernstein GA, Carroll ME, Thuras PD, Cosgrove KP, Roth ME. Caffeine dependence in teenagers. Drug Alcohol Depend. 2002;66:1–6.

23. Burgalassi A, Ramacciotti CE, Bianchi M, Coli E, Polese L, Bondi E, et al. Caffeine consumption among eating disorder patients: epidemiology, motivations, and potential of abuse. Eat Weight Disord. 2009;14:e212–e218.

24. Ciapparelli A, Paggini R, Carmassi C, Taponecco C, Consoli G, Ciampa G, et al. Patterns of caffeine consumption in psychiatric patients. an Italian study. Eur Psychiatry. 2010; 25:230–235.

25. Graham K. Reasons for consumption and heavy caffeine use: generalization of a model based on alcohol research. Addict Behav. 1988;13:209–214.

26. Heinz AJ, Kassel JD, Smith EV. Caffeine expectancy: instrument development in the rasch measurement framework. Psychol Addict Behav. 2009;23:500–511.

27. Hughes JR, Oliveto AH, Liguori A, Carpenter J, Howard T. Endorsement of DSM-IV dependence criteria among caffeine users. Drug Alcohol Depend. 1998;52:99–107.

28. Hughes JR, Oliveto AH, MacLaughlin M. Is dependence on one drug associated with dependence on other drugs? The cases of alcohol, caffeine and nicotine. Am J Addict. 2000;9:196–201.

29. Huntley ED, Juliano LM. Caffeine expectancy questionnaire (CaffEQ): construction, psychometric properties, and associations with caffeine use, caffeine dependence, and other related variables. Psychol Assess. 2012;24:592–607.

30. Jones HA, Lejuez CW. Personality correlates of caffeine dependence: the role of sensation seeking, impulsivity, and risk taking. Exp Clin Psychopharmacol. 2005;13:259–266.

31. Juliano LM, Evatt DP, Richards BD, Griffiths RR. Characterization of individuals seeking treatment for caffeine dependence. Psychol Addict Behav. 2012;26:948–954.

32. Oberstar JV, Bernstein GA, Thuras PD. Caffeine use and dependence in adolescents: one-year follow-up. J Child Adolesc Psychopharmacol. 2002;12:127–135.

33. Pallanti S, Bernardi S, Quercioli L. The shorter PROMIS questionnaire and the internet addiction scale in the assessment of multiple addictions in a high-school population: prevalence and related disability. CNS Spectr. 2006;11:966–974.

34. Strain EC, Mumford GK, Silverman K, Griffiths RR. Caffeine dependence syndrome. evidence from case histories and experimental evaluations. JAMA. 1994;272:1043–1048.

35. Striley CLW, Griffiths RR, Cottler LB. Evaluating dependence criteria for caffeine. J Caffeine Res. 2011;1:219–225.

36. Svikis DS, Berger N, Haug NA, Griffiths RR. Caffeine dependence in combination with a family history of alcoholism as a predictor of continued use of caffeine during pregnancy. Am J Psychiatry. 2005;162:2344–2351.

37. West O, Roderique-Davies G. Development and initial validation of a caffeine craving questionnaire. J Psychopharmacol. 2008;22:80–91.

DAY 3: WHY AVOID SUGAR?

1. Nicole M. Avena, Pedro Rada, and Bartley G. Hoebel. Evidence for sugar addiction: Behavioral and neurochemical effects of intermittent, excessive sugar intake. Neurosci Biobehav Rev. 2008; 32(1): 20–39. Published online 2007 May 18. doi: 10.1016/j.neubiorev.2007.04.019.

2. Hursh SR, Bauman RA. The behavioral analysis of demand. In: Green L, Kagel JH, editors. Advances in behavioral economics. Vol. 1. Norwood, NJ: Ablex; 1987. p. 117–165.

3. Campbell JD. Lifestyle, minerals and health. Med Hypotheses. 2001 Nov;57(5):521-31.

4. Swithers SE. Artificial sweeteners produce the counterintuitive effect of inducing metabolic derangements. Trends Endocrinol Metab. 2013 Sep;24(9):431-41. doi: 10.1016/j.tem.2013.05.005. Epub 2013 Jul 10.

DAY 4: WHY AVOID MEAT AND ANIMAL PRODUCTS?

1. J Am Diet Assoc. 2003 Jun;103(6):748-65. Position of the American Dietetic Association and Dietitians of Canada: Vegetarian diets. American Dietetic Association; Dietitians of Canada.

2. Bouvard, V et al. Carcinogenicity of consumption of red and processed meat. Lancet Onc, 2015(16)16:1599-1600. Available at: http://www.thelancet.com/pdfs/journals/lanonc/PIIS1470-2045(15)00444-1.pdf. Accessed July 18, 2017.

3. Castelló A, Boldo E, Pérez-Gómez B, Lope V. Adherence to the Western, Prudent and Mediterranean dietary patterns and breast cancer risk: MCC-Spain study. Maturitas. 2017 Sep;103:8-15. doi: 10.1016/j.maturitas.2017.06.020. Epub 2017 Jun 12.

4. Park SW, Kim JY, Kim YS, Lee SJ, Lee SD, Chung MK. A milk protein, casein, as a proliferation promoting factor in prostate cancer cells. World J Mens Health. 2014 Aug;32(2):76-82. doi: 10.5534/wjmh.2014.32.2.76. Epub 2014 Aug 26.

5. Koeth RA, Wang Z, Levison BS, et al. Intestinal microbiota metabolism of L-carnitine, a nutrient in red meat, promotes atherosclerosis. Nature medicine. 2013;19(5):576-585. doi:10.1038/nm.3145.

6. Ferdowsian HR, Barnard ND. Effects of plant-based diets on plasma lipids. Am J Cardiol. 2009 Oct 1;104(7):947-56. doi: 10.1016/j.amjcard.2009.05.032.

7. Virtanen HEK, Koskinen TT, Voutilainen S, Mursu J, Tuomainen TP, Kokko P, Virtanen JK.Intake of different dietary proteins and risk of type 2 diabetes in men: the Kuopio Ischaemic Heart Disease Risk Factor Study. Br J Nutr. 2017 Mar;117(6):882-893. doi: 10.1017/S0007114517000745. Epub 2017 Apr 11.

8. Shin JY, Xun P, Nakamura Y, He K. Egg consumption in relation to risk of cardiovascular disease and diabetes: a systematic review and meta-analysis. Am J Clin Nutr. 2013 Jul;98(1):146-59. doi: 10.3945/ajcn.112.051318. Epub 2013 May 15.

9. Guo J, Hobbs DA, Cockcroft JR, Elwood PC, Pickering JE, Lovegrove JA, Givens DI1,2. Association between egg consumption and cardiovascular disease events, diabetes and all-cause mortality. Eur J Nutr. 2017 Nov 2. doi: 10.1007/s00394-017-1566-0. [Epub ahead of print].

10. Hoppe C, Mølgaard C, Dalum C, Vaag A, Michaelsen KF. Differential effects of casein versus whey on fasting plasma levels of insulin, IGF-1 and IGF-1/IGFBP-3: results from a randomized 7-day supplementation study in prepubertal boys. Eur J Clin Nutr. 2009 Sep;63(9):1076-83. doi: 10.1038/ejcn.2009.34. Epub 2009 May 27.

11. Hoppe C, Mølgaard C, Juul A, Michaelsen KF. High intakes of skimmed milk, but not meat, increase serum IGF-I and IGFBP-3 in eight-year-old boys. Eur J Clin Nutr. 2004 Sep;58(9):1211-6.

ADDITIONAL REFERENCES RELATED TO MEAT CONSUMPTION

12. Craig WJ, Mangels AR; American Dietetic Association. Position of the American Dietetic Association: vegetarian diets. J Am Diet Assoc. 2009 Jul;109(7):1266-82.

13. Schwarz N, Sanna LJ, Skurnik I, Yoon C. 2007. Metacognitive experiences and the intricacies of setting people straight: Implications for debiasing and public information campaigns. Advances in experimental social psychology, Vol. 39. San Diego : Elsevier Academic Press Inc. p 127–61.

14. Schwarz N, Sanna LJ, Skurnik I, Yoon C. 2007. Metacognitive experiences and the intricacies of setting people straight: Implications for debiasing and public information campaigns. Advances in

experimental social psychology, Vol. 39. San Diego : Elsevier Academic Press Inc. p 127–61.

15. M. J. Zuidhof B. L. Schneider V. L. Carney D. R. Korver F. E. Robinson Growth, efficiency, and yield of commercial broilers from 1957, 1978, and 2005. Poultry Science, Volume 93, Issue 12, 1 December 2014, Pages 2970–2982, https://doi.org/10.3382/ps.2014-04291.

16. Lilburn M. S. Skeletal growth of commercial poultry species. Poult. Sci. 1994 vol. 7 (pg. 897-903).

17. Rath N. C., Huff G. R, Huff W. E., Balog J. M. Factors regulating bone maturity and strength in poultry. Poult. Sci., 2000 vol. 79 (pg. 1024-1032).

18. Olkowski A. A.Pathophysiology of heart failure in broiler chickens: Structural, biochemical, and molecular characteristics., Poult. Sci., 2007, vol. 86(pg. 999-1005).

19. Cheema M, Qureshi M, Havenstein G. A comparison of the immune response of a 2001 commercial broiler with a 1957 randombred broiler strain when fed representative 1957 and 2001 broiler diets., Poult. Sci., 2003, vol. 82 (pg. 1519-1529).

20. Lange IG, Daxenberger A, Schiffer B, et al. Sex hormones originating from different livestock production systems: fate and potential disrupting activity in the environment. Analytica Chimica Acta. 2002 473(1-2): 27-37.

21. J. Nichols, D & Daniel, T & Moore, Philip & R. Edwards, D & Pote, Daniel. (1997). Runoff of Estrogen Hormone 17??-Estradiol from Poultry Litter Applied to Pasture. Journal of Environmental Quality - J ENVIRON QUAL. 26. 10.2134/jeq1997.00472425002600040011x.

22. Schaum J, Schuda L, Wu C, Sears R, Ferrario J, Andrews K. A national survey of persistent, bioaccumulative, and toxic (PBT) pollutants in the United States milk supply. J Expo Anal Environ Epidemiol. 2003 May;13(3):177-86.

23. Daxenberger A, Ibarreta D, Meyer HH. Possible health impact of animal oestrogens in food. Hum Reprod Update. 2001 May-Jun;7(3):340-55.

24. Aksglaede L, Juul A, Leffers H, Skakkebaek NE, Andersson AM. The sensitivity of the child to sex steroids: possible impact of exogenous estrogens. Hum Reprod Update. 2006 Jul-Aug;12(4):341-9. Epub 2006 May 3.

25. Ganmaa D, Wang PY, Qin LQ, Hoshi K, Sato A. Is milk responsible for male reproductive disorders? Med Hypotheses. 2001 Oct;57(4):510-4.

26. Afeiche MC, Bridges ND, Williams PL, et al. Dairy intake and semen quality among men attending a fertility clinic. Fertility and sterility. 2014;101(5):1280-1287.e2. doi:10.1016/j.fertnstert.2014.02.003.

27. Afeiche M, Williams PL, Mendiola J, Gaskins AJ, Jørgensen N, Swan SH, Chavarro JE. Dairy food intake in relation to semen quality and reproductive hormone levels among physically active young men. Hum Reprod. 2013 Aug;28(8):2265-75. doi: 10.1093/humrep/det133. Epub 2013 May 12.

28. Hartmann, Sonja & Lacorn, Markus & Steinhart, Hans. (1998). Natural occurrence of steroid hormones in food. Food Chemistry. 62. 7-20. 10.1016/S0308-8146(97)00150-7.

29. Afeiche MC, Williams PL, Gaskins AJ, Mendiola J, Jørgensen N, Swan SH, Chavarro JE. Meat intake and reproductive parameters among young men. Epidemiology. 2014 May;25(3):323-30. doi: 10.1097/EDE.0000000000000092.

DAY 5: WHY AVOID ALCOHOL?

1. Gardner JD, Mouton AJ. Alcohol effects on cardiac function. Compr Physiol. 2015 Apr;5(2):791-802. doi: 10.1002/cphy.c140046.

2. Baan R, Straif K, Grosse Y, et al. Carcinogenicity of alcoholic beverages Lancet Oncology 2007;8(4):292-293.

3. IARC Working Group on the Evaluation of Carcinogenic Risks to Humans. Personal habits and indoor combustions. Volume 100 E. A review of human carcinogens. IARC Monographs on the Evaluation of Carcinogenic Risks in Humans 2012;100(Pt E):373-472.

4. Grewal P, Viswanathen VA. Liver cancer and alcohol. Clinics in Liver Disease 2012;16(4):839-850.

5. Hamajima N, Hirose K, Tajima K, et al. Alcohol, tobacco and breast cancer--collaborative reanalysis of individual data from 53 epidemiological studies, including 58,515 women with breast cancer and 95,067 women without the disease. British Journal of Cancer 2002;87(11):1234-1245.

6. Fedirko V, Tramacere I, Bagnardi V, et al. Alcohol drinking and colorectal cancer risk: an overall and dose-response meta-analysis of published studies. Annals of Oncology 2011;22(9):1958-1972.

7. NIH. National Cancer Center. Available at: https://www.cancer.gov/about-cancer/causes-prevention/risk/alcohol/alcohol-fact-sheet#q3. Last accessed: March 8, 2018.

DAY 6: WHY AVOID GLUTEN?

1. Shewry PR and Hey S. Do "ancient" wheat species differ from modern bread wheat in their contents of bioactive components? Journal of Cereal Science 2015 (65): 236-243.

2. What is Celiac Disease? https://celiac.org/celiac-disease/understanding-celiac-disease-2/what-is-celiac-disease/ Last Accessed October 22, 2017.

3. Rubio-Tapia A, Jonas F Ludvigsson JF, Brantner TL, Murray JA, Everhart JE. The Prevalence of Celiac Disease in the United States. Am J Gastroenterol 2012; 107:1538–1544; doi:10.1038/ajg.2012.219; published online 31 July 2012.

4. Vazquez-Roque MI1, Camilleri M, Smyrk T, Murray JA, et al. A controlled trial of gluten-free diet in patients with irritable bowel syndrome-diarrhea: effects on bowel frequency and intestinal function. Gastroenterology. 2013 May;144(5):903-911.e3. doi: 10.1053/j.gastro.2013.01.049. Epub 2013 Jan 25.

5. Chey WD. Symposium Report: An Evidence-Based Approach to IBS and CIC: Applying New Advances to Daily Practice. A Review of an Adjunct Clinical Symposium of the American College of Gastroenterology Meeting October 16, 2016. Gastroenterol Hepatol (N Y). 2017 Feb; 13(2 Suppl 1): 1–16.

6. Lister J, Fletcher PJ, Nobrega JN, Remington G. Behavioral effects of food-derived opioid-like peptides in rodents: Implications for schizophrenia? Pharmacol Biochem Behav. 2015 Jul;134:70-8. doi: 10.1016/j.pbb.2015.01.020. Epub 2015 Feb 7.

7. Cade R, Privette M, Fregly M, Rowland N, Sun Z, Zele V, Wagemaker H, Edelstein C1. Autism and Schizophrenia: Intestinal Disorders. Nutr Neurosci. 2000;3(1):57-72. doi: 10.1080/1028415X.2000.11747303.

8. Kim HS, Demyen MF, Mathew J, Kothari N, Feurdean M, Ahlawat SK. Obesity, Metabolic Syndrome, and Cardiovascular Risk in Gluten-Free Followers Without Celiac Disease in the United States: Results from the National Health and Nutrition Examination Survey 2009-2014. Dig Dis Sci. 2017 Apr 27. doi:

10.1007/s10620-017-4583-1. [Epub ahead of print].

9. Hamilton, C. Meditations Mini Podcast. Calm Clear Now Network. 2017. Available at: www.audioboom/channel/meditation-minis-podcast. Last accessed March 23, 2018.

ADDITIONAL REFERENCE RELATED TO GLUTEN CONSUMPTION

10. Neuman T, David K, Cooper D, Strair R. The enteric toxicity of gluten enhances graft-versus-host disease after allogeneic hematopoietic stem cell transplantation. Med Hypotheses. 2017 Jul;104:174-177. doi: 10.1016/j.mehy.2017.05.037. Epub 2017 Jun 16.

DAY 7: THE IMPORTANCE OF WATER AND SLEEP

1. Benefer MD, Corfe BM, Russell JM, Short R, Barker ME.Water intake and post-exercise cognitive performance: an observational study of long-distance walkers and runners. Eur J Nutr. 2013 Mar;52(2):617-24. doi: 10.1007/s00394-012-0364-y. Epub 2012 May 11.

2. Pross N, Demazières A, Girard N, Barnouin R, Santoro F, Chevillotte E, Klein A, Le Bellego L. Influence of progressive fluid restriction on mood and physiological markers of dehydration in women. Br J Nutr. 2013 Jan 28;109(2):313-21. doi: 10.1017/S0007114512001080. Epub 2012 Apr 13.

3. Riebl SK, Davy BM. The Hydration Equation: Update on Water Balance and Cognitive Performance. ACSM's health & fitness journal. 2013;17(6):21-28. doi:10.1249/FIT.0b013e3182a9570f.

4. Armstrong LE1, Ganio MS, Casa DJ, Lee EC, McDermott BP, Klau JF, Jimenez L, Le Bellego L, Chevillotte E, Lieberman HR. Mild dehydration affects mood in healthy young women. J Nutr. 2012 Feb;142(2):382-8. doi: 10.3945/jn.111.142000. Epub 2011 Dec 21.

5. Blau JN. Water deprivation: a new migraine precipitant. Headache. 2005 Jun;45(6):757-9.

6. Blau JN, Kell CA, Sperling JM. Water-deprivation headache: a new headache with two variants. Headache. 2004 Jan;44(1):79-83.

7. Popkin BM, D'Anci KE, Rosenberg IH. Water, Hydration and Health. Nutrition reviews. 2010;68(8):439-458. doi:10.1111/j.1753-4887.2010.00304.x.

8. Paik IY, Jeong MH, Jin HE, Kim YI, Suh AR, Cho SY, Roh HT, Jin CH, Suh SH. Fluid replacement following dehydration reduces oxidative stress during recovery. Biochem Biophys Res Commun. 2009 May 22;383(1):103-7. doi: 10.1016/j.bbrc.2009.03.135. Epub 2009 Apr 1.

9. Murakami K, Sasaki S, Okubo H, Takahashi Y, et al. Association between dietary fiber, water and magnesium intake and functional constipation among young Japanese women. European Journal of Clinical Nutrition 2007(61); 616–622. doi:10.1038/sj.ejcn.1602573.

10. Bayon V, Leger D, Gomez-Merino D, Vecchierini MF, Chennaoui M. Sleep debt and obesity. Ann Med. 2014 Aug;46(5):264-72. doi: 10.3109/07853890.2014.931103. Epub 2014 Jul 11.

11. Perkus B. Aroma Freedom Technique. Aroma Freedom International. 2016.

ADDITIONAL REFERENCE RELATED TO GLUTEN CONSUMPTION

12. Hu, FB and Patel, Sanjay. Short Sleep Duration and Weight Gain: A Systematic Review. Obesity. 2008; 16(3), 643-653.

13. Taheri S, Lin L, Austin D, Young T, Mignot E. Short Sleep Duration Is Associated with Reduced Leptin, Elevated Ghrelin, and Increased Body Mass Index. Froguel P, ed. PLoS Medicine. 2004;1(3):e62. doi:10.1371/journal.pmed.0010062.

14. Cappuccio FP, Taggart FM, Kandala N-B, et al. Meta-Analysis of Short Sleep Duration and Obesity in Children and Adults. Sleep. 2008;31(5):619-626.

15. Cappuccio FP, Cooper D, D'Elia L, Strazzullo P, Miller MA. Sleep duration predicts cardiovascular outcomes: a systematic review and meta-analysis of prospective studies. Eur Heart J. 2011 Jun;32(12):1484-92. doi: 10.1093/eurheartj/ehr007. Epub 2011 Feb 7.

16. Van Leeuwen WMA, Hublin C, Sallinen M, Härmä M, Hirvonen A, Porkka-Heiskanen T. Prolonged Sleep Restriction Affects Glucose Metabolism in Healthy Young Men. International Journal of Endocrinology. 2010; 2010:108641. doi:10.1155/2010/108641.

17. Gottlieb DJ, Punjabi NM, Newman AB, Resnick HE, Redline S, Baldwin CM, Nieto FJ. Association of sleep time with diabetes mellitus and impaired glucose tolerance. Arch Intern Med. 2005 Apr 25;165(8):863-7.

18. Kinnucan JA, Rubin DT, Ali T. Sleep and Inflammatory Bowel Disease: Exploring the Relationship Between Sleep Disturbances and Inflammation. Gastroenterology & Hepatology. 2013;9(11):718-727.

19. Ali T, Choe J, Awab A, Wagener TL, Orr WC. Sleep, immunity and inflammation in gastrointestinal disorders. World Journal of Gastroenterology : WJG. 2013;19(48):9231-9239. doi:10.3748/wjg.v19.i48.9231.

20. Robson KM1, Kiely DK, Lembo T. Development of constipation in nursing home residents. Dis Colon Rectum. 2000 Jul;43(7):940-3.

DAY 9: CHANGES IN BLOOD SUGAR AND BLOOD PRESSURE?

1. American Diabetes Association. Standards of Diabetes Care 2018. Diabetes Care. 2018(41) Supp 1. 1-172.

ADDITIONAL REFERENCES RELATED TO DIABETES AND BLOOD PRESSURE

2. 2017 ACC/AHA /AAPA/ABC/AGS/APhA/ASH/ASPC/NMA/PCNA Guideline for the Prevention, Detection, Evaluation, and Management of High Blood Pressure in Adults.

3. Balliett M, Burke JR. Changes in anthropometric measurements, body composition, blood pressure, lipid profile, and testosterone in patients participating in a low-energy dietary intervention. J Chiropr Med. 2013 Mar;12(1):3-14. doi: 10.1016/j.jcm.2012.11.003.

4. Ho CP, Yu JH, Lee TJF. Ovo-vegetarian diet is associated with lower systemic blood pressure in Taiwanese women. Public Health. 2017 Sep 25;153:70-77. doi: 10.1016/j.puhe.2017.07.032. [Epub ahead of print].

5. Kahleova H, Levin S, Barnard N. Cardio-Metabolic Benefits of Plant-Based Diets. Nutrients. 2017;9(8):848. doi:10.3390/nu9080848.

DAY 10: COMMON QUESTIONS ON PLANT BASED DIETS

1. Barrett-Connor E, Chang JC, Edelstein SL. Coffee-associated osteoporosis offset by daily milk consumption. JAMA 1994;271:280-3.

2. Massey LK, Whiting SJ. Caffeine, urinary calcium, calcium metabolism, and bone. J Nutr 1993;123:1611-4.

3. Hirsch PE, Peng TC. Effects of alcohol on calcium homeostasis and bone. In: Anderson J, Garner S, eds. Calcium and Phosphorus in Health and Disease. Boca Raton, FL: CRC Press, 1996:289-300.

4. U.S. Department of Agriculture. Results from the United States Department of Agriculture's 1994-96 Continuing Survey of Food Intakes by Individuals/Diet and Health Knowledge Survey, 1994-96.

5. D'Adamo CR, Sahin A. Soy foods and supplementation: a review of commonly perceived health benefits and risks. Altern Ther Health Med. 2014 Winter;20 Suppl 1:39-51.

6. Recommended Dietary Allowances. National Research Council (US) Subcommittee on the Tenth Edition of the Recommended Dietary Allowances. Washington (DC): National Academies Press (US); 1989. Available at: https://www.ncbi.nlm.nih.gov/books/NBK234922/. Last Accessed March 26, 2018.

7. Office of Disease Prevention and Health Prevention. Dietary Guidelines for Americans 2015-2020. 8th Ed. Available at: https://health.gov/dietaryguidelines/2015/guidelines/.

8. Clarys P, Deliens T, Huybrechts I, Peter Deriemaeker P. Comparison of Nutritional Quality of the Vegan, Vegetarian, Semi-Vegetarian, Pesco-Vegetarian and Omnivorous Diet. Nutrients. 2014 Mar; 6(3): 1318–1332. Published online 2014 Mar 24. doi: 10.3390/nu6031318.

9. Herrmann W, Schorr H, Obeid R, Geisel J. Vitamin B-12 status, particularly holotranscobalamin II and methylmalonic acid concentrations, and hyperhomocysteinemia in vegetarians. Am J Clin Nutr. 2003 Jul; 78(1):131-6.

10. Krajcovicová-Kudláčková M, Blazícek P, Kopcová J, Béderová A, et al. Homocysteine levels in vegetarians versus omnivores. Ann Nutr Metab. 2000; 44(3):135-8.

11. Majchrzak D, Singer I, Männer M, Rust P, et al. B-vitamin status and concentrations of homocysteine in Austrian omnivores, vegetarians and vegans. Ann Nutr Metab. 2006; 50(6):485-91.

12. Gilsing A.M., Growe F.L., Lioyd-Wright Z., Sanders T.A., Appleby P.N., Allen N.E., Key T.J. Serum concentrations of vitamin B12 and folate in British male omnivores, vegetarians, and vegans: Results from a cross-sectional analysis of the EPIC-Oxford cohort study. Eur. J. Clin. Nutr. 2010;64:933–939. doi: 10.1038/ejcn.2010.142.

ADDITIONAL REFERENCES RELATED TO DIABETES AND BLOOD PRESSURE

13. Committee to Review Dietary Reference Intakes for Vitamin D and Calcium, Food and Nutrition Board, Institute of Medicine. Dietary Reference Intakes for Calcium and Vitamin D. Washington, DC: National Academy Press, 2010.

14. Institute of Agriculture and Natural Resources. Food Allergy Research and Resource Program. Allergenic Foods and their Allergens.

DAY 11: THE ENVIRONMENT

1. Hallock B. To make a burger, first you need 660 gallons of water. Los Angeles Times 2014 January 27. Available at: http://www.latimes.com/food/dailydish/la-dd-gallons-of-water-to-make-a-burger-20140124-story.html.

2. Schaum J, Schuda L, Wu C, Sears R, Ferrario J, Andrews K. A national survey of persistent, bioaccumulative, and toxic (PBT) pollutants in the United States milk supply. J Expo Anal Environ Epidemiol. 2003 May;13(3):177-86.

3. Hellberg, R. S., DeWitt, C. A. M. and Morrissey, M. T. (2012), Risk-Benefit Analysis of Seafood Consumption: A Review. Comprehensive Reviews in Food Science and Food Safety, 11: 490–517. doi:10.1111/j.1541-4337.2012.00200.x.

4. Yasumoto T, Murata M. 1993. Marine toxins. Chem Rev 93(5):1897–909.

5. Plessi M, Bertelli D, Monzani A. 2001. Mercury and selenium content in selected seafood. J Food Comp Anal 14(5):461–7.

6. Storelli MM, Giacominelli-Stuffler R, Storelli A, Marcotrigiano GO. 2003. Polychlorinated biphenyls in seafood: contamination levels and human dietary exposure. Food Chem 82(3):491–6.

7. Iwamoto M, Ayers T, Mahon BE, Swerdlow DL. 2010. Epidemiology of seafood-associated infections in the United States. Clin Microbiol Rev 23(2):399–411.

8. Gunderson EL. 1995. Dietary intakes of pesticides, selected elements, and other chemicals: FDA total diet study, June 1984-April 1986. J AOAC Intl 78(4):910–21.

9. Watanabe C, Satoh H. 1996. Evolution of our understanding of methylmercury as a health threat. Environ Health Perspect 104(Suppl 2):367–79.

10. Juhlshamn K, Andersen A, Ringdal O, Morkore J. 1987. Trace elements intake in the Faroe Islands: I. Element levels in edible parts of pilot whales (globicephalus meleanus). Sci Total Environ 65:53–62.

11. Oken E, Kleinman KP, Berland WE, Simon SR, Rich-Edwards JW, Gillman MW. 2003. Decline in fish consumption among pregnant women after a national mercury advisory. Obstet Gynecol 102(2):346–351.

ADDITIONAL REFERENCES RELATED TO DIABETES AND BLOOD PRESSURE

12. Rosi A, Mena P, Pellegrini N, et al. Environmental impact of omnivorous, ovo-lacto-vegetarian, and vegan diet. Scientific Reports. 2017;7:6105. doi:10.1038/s41598-017-06466-8.

13. Stehfest E. Diet: Food choices for health and planet. Nature. 2014 Nov 27; 515(7528):501-2.

14. Joyce A, Dixon S, Comfort J, Hallett J. Reducing the environmental impact of dietary choice: perspectives from a behavioural and social change approach. J Environ Public Health. 2012; 2012():978672.

15. Hodson G, Earle M. Appetite. 2017 Aug 30;120:75-81. doi: 10.1016/j.appet.2017.08.027. [Epub ahead of print] Conservatism predicts lapses from vegetarian/vegan diets to meat consumption (through lower social justice concerns and social support).

16. Liu, Junguo, Yang, Hong, & Savenije, H.H.G. China's move to higher-meat diet hits water security. Nature 454.397 (2008). doi: 10.1038/454397a.

DAY 14: WHY AVOID MEAT. PART 2

1. Centers for Disease Control. Foodborne Germs and Illnesses. https://www.cdc.gov/foodsafety/foodborne-germs.html.

2. Daxenberger A, Ibarreta D, Meyer HH. Possible health impact of animal oestrogens in food. Hum Reprod Update. 2001 May-Jun;7(3):340-55.

3. Aksglaede L, Juul A, Leffers H, Skakkebaek NE, Andersson AM. The sensitivity of the child to sex steroids: possible impact of exogenous estrogens. Hum Reprod Update. 2006 Jul-Aug;12(4):341-9. Epub 2006 May 3.

4. Hartmann, Sonja & Lacorn, Markus & Steinhart, Hans. (1998). Natural occurrence of steroid hormones in food. Food Chemistry. 62. 7-20. 10.1016/S0308-8146(97)00150-7.

5. Afeiche M, Williams PL, Mendiola J, Gaskins AJ, Jørgensen N, Swan SH, Chavarro JE. Dairy food intake in relation to semen quality and reproductive hormone levels among physically active young men. Hum Reprod. 2013 Aug;28(8):2265-75. doi: 10.1093/humrep/det133. Epub 2013 May 12.

6. Afeiche MC, Williams PL, Gaskins AJ, Mendiola J, Jørgensen N, Swan SH, Chavarro JE. Meat intake and reproductive parameters among young men. Epidemiology. 2014 May;25(3):323-30. doi: 10.1097/EDE.0000000000000092.

7. Lange IG, Daxenberger A, Schiffer B, et al. Sex hormones originating from different livestock production systems: fate and potential disrupting activity in the environment. Analytica Chimica Acta. 2002 473(1-2): 27-37.

8. J. Nichols, D & Daniel, T & Moore, Philip & R. Edwards, D & Pote, Daniel. (1997). Runoff of Estrogen Hormone 17??-Estradiol from Poultry Litter Applied to Pasture. Journal of Environmental Quality - J ENVIRON QUAL. 26. 10.2134/jeq1997.00472425002600040011x.

9. Afeiche MC, Bridges ND, Williams PL, et al. Dairy intake and semen quality among men attending a fertility clinic. Fertility and sterility. 2014;101(5):1280-1287.e2. doi:10.1016/j.fertnstert.2014.02.003.

10. Lawton, S. Implanting Beef Cattle. Bulletin 1302. Available at: http://extension.uga.edu/publications/detail.html?number=B1302#Table1.

11. M. J. Zuidhof B. L. Schneider V. L. Carney D. R. Korver F. E. Robinson Growth, efficiency, and yield of commercial broilers from 1957, 1978, and 2005. Poultry Science, Volume 93, Issue 12, 1 December 2014, Pages 2970–2982, https://doi.org/10.3382/ps.2014-04291.

12. Lilburn M. S. Skeletal growth of commercial poultry species. Poult. Sci. 1994 vol. 7 (pg. 897-903).

13. Rath N. C., Huff G. R, Huff W. E., Balog J. M. Factors regulating bone maturity and strength in poultry. Poult. Sci., 2000 vol. 79 (pg. 1024-1032).

14. Olkowski A. A Pathophysiology of heart failure in broiler chickens: Structural, biochemical, and molecular characteristics., Poult. Sci., 2007, vol. 86(pg. 999-1005).

15. Cheema M, Qureshi M, Havenstein G. A comparison of the immune response of a 2001 commercial broiler with a 1957 randombred broiler strain when fed representative 1957 and 2001 broiler diets., Poult. Sci., 2003, vol. 82 (pg. 1519-1529).

DAY 15: MINDFUL EATING

1. Roth, G. Women, Food and God: An Unexpected Path to Almost Everything. 2011. Simon & Schuster Ltd. London, UK.

DAY 17: CASTOR OIL PACK

1. Arslan GG, Eser I. An examination of the effect of castor oil packs on constipation in the elderly. Complement Ther Clin Pract. 2011 Feb;17(1):58-62.
2. Tunaru S, Althoff TF, Nüsing RM, Diener M, Offermanns S. Castor oil induces laxation and uterus contraction via ricinoleic acid activating prostaglandin EP3 receptors. Proceedings of the National Academy of Sciences of the United States of America. 2012;109(23):9179-9184. doi:10.1073/pnas.1201627109.

ADDITIONAL REFERENCES RELATED TO CASTOR OIL PACKS

3. Vieira C, Evangelista S, Cirillo R, Lippi A, Maggi CA, Manzini S (2000). "Effect of ricinoleic acid in acute and subchronic experimental models of inflammation". Mediators Inflamm. 9 (5): 223–8. doi:1080/09629350020025737. PMC1781768. PMID 11200362.
4. Grady H. Immunomodulation Through Castor Oil Packs Journal of Naturopathic Medicine. Volume 7, Number 1 1999.
5. Duke, JA. Ricinus Communis. Ricinus Communis L. 1998. Web. 9 Apr. 2013.
6. Marwat SK, Rehman F, Khan EA, Baloch MS, Sadiq M, Ullah I, Javaria S, Shaheen S. Review - Ricinus cmmunis - Ethnomedicinal uses and pharmacological activities. Pak J Pharm Sci. 2017 Sep;30(5): 1815-1827.

DAY 18: GALL BLADDER CLEANSE

1. Pitchford, P. Healing with Whole Foods. 3rd ed. 2002. North Atlantic Books. Berkeley, California.
2. Key TJ, Davey GK, Appleby PN. Health benefits of a vegetarian diet. Proc Nutr Soc. 1999 May;58(2):271-5.

ADDITIONAL REFERENCES RELATED TO CASTOR OIL PACKS

3. Dwyer JT. Health aspects of vegetarian diets. Am J Clin Nutr. 1988 Sep;48(3 Suppl):712-38.

DAY 19: COFFEE ENEMA

1. Gerson M. The cure of advanced cancer by diet therapy: a summary of 30 years of clinical experimentation. Physiol Chem Phys. 1978;10(5):449-64.

2. Cassileth B. Gerson regimen. Oncology (Williston Park). 2010 Feb;24(2):201.

3. Sashiyama H, Hamahata Y, Matsuo K, Akagi K, Tsutsumi O, Nakajima Y, Takaishi Y, Takase Y, Arai T, Hoshino T, Tazawa A, Fu KI, Tsujinaka Y. Rectal burn caused by hot-water coffee enema. Gastrointest Endosc. 2008 Nov;68(5):1008; discussion 1009. doi: 10.1016/j.gie.2008.04.017. Epub 2008 Jul 26.

4. Eisele, J, Reay, D. Deaths related to coffee enemas. JAMA 1980. 244 (14): 1608–1609.

ADDITIONAL REFERENCES RELATED TO COFFEE ENEMAS

5. Lee, M. The Study of Enema Therapy as One of the Detoxification Therapy. Journal of Oriental Neuropsychiatry. 2004; 15(2): 23-36.

6. Lam LKT, Sparnins VL and Wattenberg LW. Effects of Derivatives of Kahweol and Cafestol on the Activity of Glutathione S-Transferase in Mice. J Med Chem. 1987; 30(8):1399-1403.

7. Lam LKT, Sparnins VL and Wattenberg LW. Isolation and identification of kahweol palmitate and cafestol palmitate as active constituents of green coffee beans that enhance glutathione S-transferase activity in the mouse. Cancer Res. 1982;42:1193-1198.

8. Sparnins VL and Wattenberg LW. Enhancement of glutathione S-transferase activity of the mouse forestomach by inhibitors of benzo[a]pyrene-induced neoplasia of forestomach. J Natl Cancer Inst. 1981;66:769-771.

9. Lechner P. A reply to Saul Green's critique of the rationale for cancer treatment with coffee enemas and diet: cafestol derived from beverage coffee increases bile production in rats; and coffee enemas and diet ameliorate human cancer pain in Stages I and II. Available at: http://gerson-research.org/research/reply-saul-greens-critique-rationale-cancer-treatment-coffee-enemas-diet-cafestol-derived-beverage-coffee-increases-bile-production-rats-coffee-enemas/.

10. Margolin KA, Green MR. Polymicrobial enteric septicemia from coffee enemas. West J Med. 1984 Mar;140(3):460.

DAY 21: GOALS REFLECTION: DEAR PAST ME

1. Hamilton, C. Meditations Mini Podcast. Calm Clear Now Network. 2017. Available at: www.audioboom/channel/meditation-minis-podcast. Last accessed March 23, 2018.

DISCLAIMER

The Clean Slate Cleanse is a 21-Day program that eliminates meat and animal products, caffeine, sugar, wheat and gluten, and alcohol. This is a vegan cleanse. The statements in this book have not been evaluated by the Food and Drug Administration.

You should consult your physician or other health care professional before starting any cleanse to determine if it is right for your needs. This is particularly true if you (or your family) have a history of disease or if you are pregnant or nursing. Do not change your diet if your physician recommends against it.

There is a risk that blood sugar and blood pressures may be lowered. Report these to your physician immediately. If you are taking medications to treat diabetes or hypertension, you must check your blood sugar and blood pressure regularly.

You may experience withdrawal symptoms from caffeine or sugar including headache, tiredness, or inability to focus. These generally resolve in 2-3 days. If symptoms persist, report to your physician.

Withdrawal from alcohol addiction can be severe and life-threatening. If you experience cravings, anxiety, shakiness, rapid heart rate, vomiting, itching, delirium, or see things that aren't there, report to a physician immediately.

If you are in the United States and experience a medical emergency, call your health care professional, or 911, immediately. If you have food allergies, we have a wide variety of options and substitutions. If you experience any symptoms of allergy, including itching, swelling, redness, or swelling of the throat, report to a physician immediately or call 911.

The Clean Slate Cleanse does not cure diabetes, high blood pressure, or any other disease or illness. Individual results may vary. Weight loss is not typical. There is no guarantee that you will lose weight with this program.

Additional caution should be exercised with the complimentary cleanses: the castor oil pack, coffee enema, and gallbladder flush. Follow instructions closely and discuss with a physician before completing additional cleanses.

You are entering this program at your own risk. The responsibility for the consequences of your use of any suggestion or procedure described in this book lies not with Lindsey Kay Elmore, LLC.

ACKNOWLEDGEMENTS

To the #cleanslaters, the changes you go through on this cleanse inspire me to be better and inspired me to write this book. I'm so grateful that you follow along @cleanslatecleanse on Instagram and @thecleanslatecleanse on Facebook.

To the unwavering support of Justin Anderson, Shelbi Kribell, Jen McCraw and Julie Folger. This book would not exist without you.

BIOGRAPHY

Dr. Lindsey Elmore is a small-town girl with a big dream. She is a speaker, wellness advocate, and author. What Lindsey does well is take complicated science information and make it simple. What Dr. Elmore does well is analyze data to inform her presentations. Originally trained as a chemist and then a clinical pharmacist, she now crafts memorable, relatable science stories about essential oils, herbs, and foods.

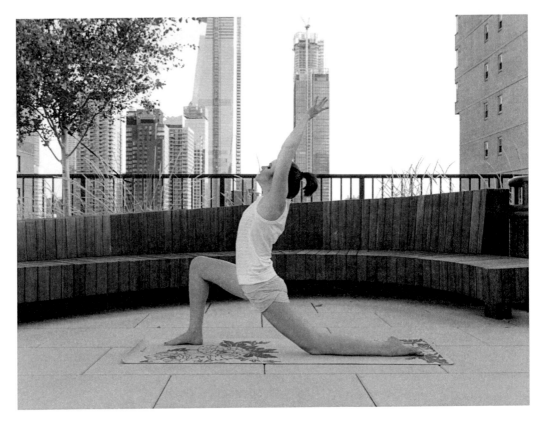

During her preteens and teenage years, she struggled with bulimia. She became a vegetarian for all the wrong reasons. As a means of restriction instead of as a vehicle to optimal health. She has been off and on gluten-free, vegan for many years, and has a deep love of cooking, especially vegetables. Though she is now a city dweller, she spent years with her family tending to gardens as a child and to her own garden as an adult. She is a huge advocate of homegrown food, and staunchly opposed to genetic modification for the purpose of resistance to herbicides and insertion of terminator genes. No to monoculture of foods.

She obtained an undergraduate degree in chemistry from the University of Alabama Birmingham and a doctorate in pharmacy from the University of California San Francisco. She completed her first-year post-doctoral residency in pharmacy practice at Princeton Baptist Medical Center in Birmingham, AL and her second-year specialty residency in ambulatory care at New Hanover Regional Medical Center in Wilmington, NC. She is a Board-Certified Pharmacotherapy Specialist and licensed to practice in three states. She believes that the pharmacist is healthcare's most underutilized resource. Not only do pharmacists know medicines, they teach patients how to optimize their medicines. If your pharmacist misses either of these traits, break away from the chain and go to support a local, independent pharmacy. Please vote for leaders who support expansion of pharmacy practice acts. As has been demonstrated in North Carolina, pharmacists improve disease state control and save health care dollars when they are granted authority to manage medication.

Dr. Elmore has spoken on 5 continents to local, state, national and international audiences. Her

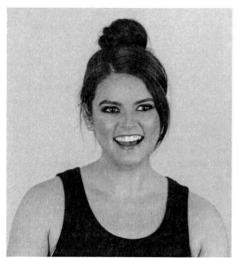

presentation materials have been translated into more than 20 languages. She is published in a wide variety of pharmacy and medical journals and has a long history of service with the American Society of Health System Pharmacists. She served as a visiting scholar at the University of Zambia, Department of Medicine and provided direct patient care in family medicine, community pharmacy, and inpatient care for years before changing course to embrace health care instead of sick care.

Dr. Elmore is passionate about mindful wellness. She is a Certified 200 hr. yoga instructor, an Aroma Yoga® Instructor, an Aroma Freedom Technique Instructor, and an advocate of whole foods as medicine. She has been a patient of Chinese medicine and acupuncture for over a decade and blends Eastern and Western concepts of health in all her teaching.

Dr. Elmore's teaching has inspired hundreds of thousands of people to take ownership of their health and wellness, and the group grows every day. Join her on her journey: on Instagram @lindseyelmore and @cleanslatecleanse on Facebook at www.facebook.com/lindseyelmore and www.facebook.com/thecleanslatecleanse and online at www.lindseyelmore.com.

In her spare time, Dr. Elmore enjoys giving thanks, swimming in oceans, rivers and streams, singing, dancing alone in her apartment, and watching her brother play professional baseball. She currently resides in New York City.

FOR MORE INFO VISIT

www.lindseyelmore.com

FOLLOW ON FACEBOOK & INSTAGRAM

@lindseyelmore